Overcoming Common Problems

The Fibromyalgia Healing Diet

Third edition

CHRISTINE CRAGGS-HINTON

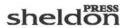

sheldon PRESS

First published in Great Britain in 2001

Sheldon Press
36 Causton Street
London SW1P 4ST
www.sheldonpress.co.uk

Reprinted twice
Second edition published 2008
Reprinted once
Third edition published 2014

British Library Cataloguing-in-Publication Data
A catalogue record for this book is available from the British Library

ISBN 978–1–84709–349–3
eBook ISBN 978–1–84709–350–9

Typeset by Fakenham Prepress Solutions, Fakenham, Norfolk NR21 8NN
First printed in Great Britain by Ashford Colour Press
Subsequently digitally reprinted in Great Britain

eBook by Fakenham Prepress Solutions, Fakenham, Norfolk NR21 8NN

Produced on paper from sustainable forests

The Fibromyalgia Healing Diet

Christine Craggs-Hinton, mother of three, followed a career in the Civil Service until, in 1991, she developed fibromyalgia, a chronic pain condition. Christine took up writing for therapeutic reasons and, in the next few years, produced more than a dozen health-related self-help books for Sheldon Press. She also wrote for the Fibromyalgia Association UK and the UK Fibromyalgia magazine called *FaMily*. In 2007 Christine and her husband moved to the Canary Islands where she worked as the agony aunt and health writer for a local newspaper. Christine died in 2013.

C333648482

Overcoming Common Problems Series

Selected titles

A full list of titles is available from Sheldon Press,
36 Causton Street, London SW1P 4ST and on our website at
www.sheldonpress.co.uk

101 Questions to Ask Your Doctor
Dr Tom Smith

Asperger Syndrome in Adults
Dr Ruth Searle

Assertiveness: Step by step
Dr Windy Dryden and Daniel Constantinou

Birth Over 35
Sheila Kitzinger

Body Language: What you need to know
David Cohen

Breast Cancer: Your treatment choices
Dr Terry Priestman

Bulimia, Binge-eating and their Treatment
Professor J. Hubert Lacey, Dr Bryony Bamford
and Amy Brown

The Cancer Survivor's Handbook
Dr Terry Priestman

**Chronic Fatigue Syndrome: What you need
to know about CFS/ME**
Dr Megan A. Arroll

The Chronic Pain Diet Book
Neville Shone

Cider Vinegar
Margaret Hills

Coeliac Disease: What you need to know
Alex Gazzola

**Coping Successfully with Chronic Illness: Your
healing plan**
Neville Shone

Coping Successfully with Pain
Neville Shone

Coping Successfully with Prostate Cancer
Dr Tom Smith

Coping Successfully with Shyness
Margaret Oakes, Professor Robert Bor
and Dr Carina Eriksen

Coping Successfully with Ulcerative Colitis
Peter Cartwright

Coping Successfully with Varicose Veins
Christine Craggs-Hinton

Coping Successfully with Your Hiatus Hernia
Dr Tom Smith

Coping When Your Child Has Cerebral Palsy
Jill Eckersley

Coping with Anaemia
Dr Tom Smith

Coping with Asthma in Adults
Mark Greener

**Coping with Birth Trauma
and Postnatal Depression**
Lucy Jolin

Coping with Bronchitis and Emphysema
Dr Tom Smith

Coping with Candida
Shirley Trickett

Coping with Chemotherapy
Dr Terry Priestman

Coping with Chronic Fatigue
Trudie Chalder

Coping with Difficult Families
Dr Jane McGregor and Tim McGregor

Coping with Diverticulitis
Peter Cartwright

Coping with Drug Problems in the Family
Lucy Jolin

Coping with Dyspraxia
Jill Eckersley

Coping with Early-onset Dementia
Jill Eckersley

**Coping with Eating Disorders and
Body Image**
Christine Craggs-Hinton

Coping with Epilepsy
Dr Pamela Crawford and Fiona Marshall

Coping with Gout
Christine Craggs-Hinton

Coping with Guilt
Dr Windy Dryden

Coping with Headaches and Migraine
Alison Frith

Coping with Heartburn and Reflux
Dr Tom Smith

Coping with Life after Stroke
Dr Mareeni Raymond

**Coping with Life's Challenges: Moving on
from adversity**
Dr Windy Dryden

Coping with Liver Disease
Mark Greener

Overcoming Common Problems Series

Coping with Manipulation: When others blame you for their feelings
Dr Windy Dryden

Coping with Memory Problems
Dr Sallie Baxendale

Coping with Obsessive Compulsive Disorder
Professor Kevin Gournay, Rachel Piper
and Professor Paul Rogers

Coping with Phobias and Panic
Professor Kevin Gournay

Coping with Polycystic Ovary Syndrome
Christine Craggs-Hinton

Coping with the Psychological Effects of Cancer
Professor Robert Bor, Dr Carina Eriksen
and Ceilidh Stapelkamp

Coping with Radiotherapy
Dr Terry Priestman

Coping with Schizophrenia
Professor Kevin Gournay and Debbie Robson

Coping with Snoring and Sleep Apnoea
Jill Eckersley

Coping with Stomach Ulcers
Dr Tom Smith

Coping with Suicide
Maggie Helen

Coping with Thyroid Disease
Mark Greener

Coping with Type 2 Diabetes
Susan Elliot-Wright

Depressive Illness: The curse of the strong
Dr Tim Cantopher

The Diabetes Healing Diet
Mark Greener and Christine Craggs-Hinton

Dying for a Drink
Dr Tim Cantopher

The Empathy Trap: Understanding antisocial personalities
Dr Jane McGregor and Tim McGregor

Epilepsy: Complementary and alternative treatments
Dr Sallie Baxendale

The Fibromyalgia Healing Diet
Christine Craggs-Hinton

Fibromyalgia: Your treatment guide
Christine Craggs-Hinton

A Guide to Anger Management
Mary Hartley

Hay Fever: How to beat it
Dr Paul Carson

The Heart Attack Survival Guide
Mark Greener

Helping Children Cope with Grief
Rosemary Wells

Helping Elderly Relatives
Jill Eckersley

The Holistic Health Handbook
Mark Greener

How to Beat Worry and Stress
Dr David Delvin

How to Come Out of Your Comfort Zone
Dr Windy Dryden

How to Develop Inner Strength
Dr Windy Dryden

How to Eat Well When You Have Cancer
Jane Freeman

How to Live with a Control Freak
Barbara Baker

How to Lower Your Blood Pressure: And keep it down
Christine Craggs-Hinton

How to Manage Chronic Fatigue
Christine Craggs-Hinton

How to Stop Worrying
Dr Frank Tallis

The IBS Healing Plan
Theresa Cheung

The Irritable Bowel Diet Book
Rosemary Nicol

Let's Stay Together: A guide to lasting relationships
Jane Butterworth

Living with Angina
Dr Tom Smith

Living with Autism
Fiona Marshall

Living with Bipolar Disorder
Dr Neel Burton

Living with Complicated Grief
Professor Craig A. White

Living with Crohn's Disease
Dr Joan Gomez

Living with Eczema
Jill Eckersley

Living with Fibromyalgia
Christine Craggs-Hinton

Living with Gluten Intolerance
Jane Feinmann

Living with IBS
Nuno Ferreira and David T. Gillanders

Living with Loss and Grief
Julia Tugendhat

Living with Osteoporosis
Dr Joan Gomez

Overcoming Common Problems Series

Living with a Stoma
Professor Craig A. White

Living with Tinnitus and Hyperacusis
Dr Laurence McKenna, Dr David Baguley
and Dr Don McFerran

Losing a Parent
Fiona Marshall

**Making Sense of Trauma: How to tell
your story**
Dr Nigel C. Hunt and Dr Sue McHale

Menopause in Perspective
Philippa Pigache

Motor Neurone Disease: A family affair
Dr David Oliver

The Multiple Sclerosis Diet Book
Tessa Buckley

Natural Treatments for Arthritis
Christine Craggs-Hinton

Overcome Your Fear of Flying
Professor Robert Bor, Dr Carina Eriksen
and Margaret Oakes

Overcoming Anorexia
Professor J. Hubert Lacey, Christine Craggs-Hinton
and Kate Robinson

Overcoming Emotional Abuse
Susan Elliot-Wright

Overcoming Fear: With mindfulness
Deborah Ward

**Overcoming Gambling: A guide for problem
and compulsive gamblers**
Philip Mawer

Overcoming Hurt
Dr Windy Dryden

Overcoming Jealousy
Dr Windy Dryden

Overcoming Loneliness
Alice Muir

**Overcoming Panic and Related
Anxiety Disorders**
Margaret Hawkins

Overcoming Procrastination
Dr Windy Dryden

Overcoming Shyness and Social Anxiety
Dr Ruth Searle

Overcoming Stress
Professor Robert Bor, Dr Carina Eriksen
and Dr Sara Chaudry

Overcoming Worry and Anxiety
Dr Jerry Kennard

**The Pain Management Handbook: Your
personal guide**
Neville Shone

The Panic Workbook
Dr Carina Eriksen, Professor Robert Bor
and Margaret Oakes

**Physical Intelligence: How to take charge
of your weight**
Dr Tom Smith

Reducing Your Risk of Dementia
Dr Tom Smith

**Self-discipline: How to get it and how to
keep it**
Dr Windy Dryden

The Self-Esteem Journal
Alison Waines

Sinusitis: Steps to healing
Dr Paul Carson

Stammering: Advice for all ages
Renée Byrne and Louise Wright

Stress-related Illness
Dr Tim Cantopher

Ten Steps to Positive Living
Dr Windy Dryden

**Therapy for Beginners: How to get the best
out of counselling**
Professor Robert Bor, Sheila Gill and
Anne Stokes

Think Your Way to Happiness
Dr Windy Dryden and Jack Gordon

**Tranquillizers and Antidepressants: When to
take them, how to stop**
Professor Malcolm Lader

**Transforming Eight Deadly Emotions
into Healthy Ones**
Dr Windy Dryden

The Traveller's Good Health Guide
Dr Ted Lankester

Treating Arthritis Diet Book
Margaret Hills

Treating Arthritis: The drug-free way
Margaret Hills and Christine Horner

**Treating Arthritis: More ways to a
drug-free life**
Margaret Hills

Treating Arthritis: The supplements guide
Julia Davies

Understanding Obsessions and Compulsions
Dr Frank Tallis

Understanding Traumatic Stress
Dr Nigel Hunt and Dr Sue McHale

**Understanding Yourself and Others: Practical
ideas from the world of coaching**
Bob Thomson

When Someone You Love Has Dementia
Susan Elliot-Wright

**When Someone You Love Has Depression:
A handbook for family and friends**
Barbara Baker

Contents

Acknowledgements		ix
Foreword		xi
Preface		xiii
Introduction		xv

Part 1

1	What it means to have fibromyalgia	3
2	Basic considerations for health	7
3	Necessary foods	16
4	Why diet is important in treating fibromyalgia	27
5	Essential nutrients	30
6	Substances to avoid	50
7	On your way to better health – the detoxification programme	62

Part 2: Healing recipes

Essential basics	85
Breakfasts	89
Soups	91
Main meals	95
Salads	121
Desserts	124
Cakes and biscuits	127
Snacks	132
Breads	134
Drinks	136

References	142
Useful addresses	143
Further reading	147
Index	149

This book is dedicated to my dearly loved husband David – the most selfless man I have ever been lucky enough to meet. I have never felt truly alone with my illness, for he has always been there at my side, fighting my battles with me, searching for answers and managing to make me smile, even when it looked like it would take a miracle to do so! David has been an enormous help in the preparation of this book, for he has tested every single recipe, even coming up with a few tasty recipes of his own.

I would like to mention my three boys, too – Mark, James and Matthew Earley. They are wonderful, caring young men I am incredibly proud to call my own. Thank you, boys, for being so good to your old mum!

Acknowledgements

I would like to say special thanks to:

Steve Taylor, a nutritionist, who has been a terrific help to me during the writing of this book. Steve has been with me every step of the way, providing valuable information and thoroughly checking my facts.

Mavis Bannan, my very close friend, who recently died after a long struggle with cancer, for, despite her illness, she generously offered her help and support in all my ventures and throughout the worst days of my own illness – I will never forget her enormous kindness and bravery.

Acknowledgements

Foreword

There is an incredible power in each of us. It is the power and capacity to heal ourselves. Our bodies have an innate self-repair mechanism that we somehow have lost or hidden away in the corner of our stress-filled lives. We fail to take responsibility for our own illnesses and relinquish them to our modern-day doctors with their strong and often toxic drugs, expecting to take a few tablets for that 'quick fix', so that we can get back on the treadmill of life.

In the past, before the advent of 'conventional' medicine, people would use the extracts of plants, herbs, shrubs and trees to heal their ailments, each having specific properties for specific conditions. The properties of natural substances have been known and used for thousands of years. Ancient civilizations have documented evidence of their use. And what do these natural substances contain – vitamins, minerals, bioflavonoids, phyto-nutrients, etc. In other words, nutrition.

We need 13 vitamins, 22 minerals, 8 amino acids and 2 essential fatty acids to sustain life. The elimination of any one of these nutrients from the diet will ultimately result in death, it's as simple as that! Repeated studies have shown that we do not achieve the RDAs for many of the above nutrients and the RDA is the *minimum* amount required to avoid disease, not the optimum level to achieve good health.

Good nutrition is one of the cornerstones of health. However, under-ripened and overprocessed foods, with the use of chemical pesticides and fertilizers, have denatured our foods by an average of 50 per cent over the last 60 years. It's no wonder our health service cannot cope with the numbers of ill people our food industry is producing. Heart attacks, strokes, diabetes, arthritis, osteoporosis and even cancer have been linked to nutritional deficiencies. In the words of Linus Pauling, twice Nobel Prize winner for his research into vitamin C, 'Virtually all illness and disease can be attributed to a mineral deficiency.'

The food industry spends millions of pounds each year on slick advertising and marketing campaigns, telling us how good their products are. Well, I am afraid you can't beat foods that are fresh, unadulterated, unpackaged, unprocessed and hopefully organic. If you see labels such as long life, no added sugar, low fat or some other 'benefit', then please ignore this food. Its benefit will be far outweighed by some negative factor. Sugar is replaced with artificial sweeteners, for which studies have questioned the carcinogenic potential. Low fat usually means that sugar has been added to improve taste (fat tastes nice). Educate yourself about food labels and always read them. Contact a nutritional organization for help in this area.

In this book you will find some very practical advice on healthy eating. Own 'your' responsibility for 'your' illness and unleash your body's instinctive healing powers. Reclaim your health by choosing the foods recommended in this book and using correct nutritional supplements that are designed to be therapeutic, not just for general use. Put yourself in the driving seat.

Good health.

Steve Taylor, BANT Raw NCDip
Member of the British Association of
Nutritional Therapists (BANT)

P.S. Always remember that what works for one person may not work for another. Therefore, I also recommend you seek out a competent nutritional practitioner who will work closely with you to achieve your health goals.

Preface

As with Christine's first book, *Living with Fibromyalgia* (third edition, Sheldon Press, 2014), this book has been very well researched and is presented in a way that is logical and easy to understand. Many books tell you what to eat, but few explain why, which is what Christine has done here.

In the book, we are even forgiven the occasional lapse from the recommended diet when we perhaps eat out or go on holiday. Many books are too stringent and narrow in their recommendations, whereas this book would be equally suitable for people who don't have fibromyalgia, who would benefit from the common-sense approach here to topics such as additives, preservatives and so on.

Definitely a book to keep handy in the kitchen!

Bob Stewart, former Chair,
Fibromyalgia Association UK

Preface.

Introduction

Although much research has been conducted into fibromyalgia in recent years, no truly curative treatment has been found. We know that painkillers can temporarily dampen the pain sensation and that certain antidepressants can reduce the intensity of the pain, but neither of these has the effect we truly desire – that of instigating healing.

Eating certain ordinary foods can, however, promote great improvements in fibromyalgia. It can gradually normalize the body's systems and help the body to repair itself, with the possibility of eliminating the pain as well as the other myriad symptoms, restoring us to a more active, fulfilling life.

Using the guidelines set out in my previous book, *Living with Fibromyalgia* (third edition, Sheldon Press, 2014), I was able to make vast improvements to my own condition. After being bedbound and in terrible pain for several years, I found that gentle exercise, wiser use of medication, certain complementary therapies and pain and stress management techniques set me on the road to better health. I felt I was getting my life back – a different life than before my illness, I admit, but one in which real hope was beginning to flourish for the first time in years. I became able to manage my reduced levels of pain, accept my limitations and even to find the confidence to take on new challenges, such as writing my first book. At the same time, I was not happy to stay as I was. That there was more help for me and other people with fibromyalgia out there somewhere was something I was sure of – I just had to keep searching until I found it.

Then, a few months later, at one of my local fibromyalgia support group meetings, we were introduced to Steve Taylor, a nutritionist. Steve – an enthusiastic, knowledgeable young man – informed us that it is possible to redress the many bodily imbalances in fibromyalgia by following a particular diet. He said it was possible for us to heal ourselves, using food. I knew instantly that this was what I had been searching for, so wasted no time in making the recommended improvements to my diet.

The 'fibromyalgia healing diet' has become the most effective treatment I could have wished for – the foods used being, overall, no more expensive than the foods I was used to. I learned how to resolve the many nutritional deficiencies found in fibromyalgia; I learned about the toxic build-up caused, among other things, by food additives and preservatives; I learned how to follow a detoxification programme to eliminate these toxins from my body, and many more things. It is not a calorie-counting diet, and I was relieved to find there are usually appetizing substitute foods that I can eat in place of those that have to be eliminated. It is largely a matter of checking labels at the supermarket and stopping off occasionally at the local healthfood shop.

I soon found I was enjoying my new regime, making sure to maximize its effects by taking exercise and a little fresh air every day. More exciting, however, was the fact that, after a couple of months, my irritable bowel syndrome started to settle down, my pain levels were dropping sharply, and I had more energy than I had had in years. The other symptoms tied in with my fibromyalgia were becoming less of a problem, too – and all because of my changed diet!

As I continue to eat the right foods and take the recommended nutritional supplements, I continue to improve. I cannot begin to describe how it feels to be so much better. It feels like I have been given a second chance at my life. Admittedly, I have to build up my strength now, quite substantially, by exercising, but, to be able to exercise and not feel shattered and in pain afterwards is wonderful in itself.

I must stress here that just as no two people with fibromyalgia suffer identical symptoms, so no two people will respond in the same way to the diet recommended in this book. Some of you may find that, in time, your symptoms disappear completely; others may experience a less dramatic effect. However, I can assure you that there will be a change in your condition for the better, and that it will be at a fundamental level, for the diet treats the cause of the disease, not just the symptoms.

Our bodies are powerful self-generating organisms. When provided with the right fuels, they start to heal themselves. The fibromyalgia healing diet stimulates healing of all the body's systems, allowing those systems to function in the way they were intended.

Thy food shall be thy remedy

Hippocrates, the father of modern medicine

This book sets out the recommended foods and nutritional supplements, as well as the substances to avoid. The 21-day detoxification programme is described in later pages.

Before you start

The diet described in this book should only be followed with your doctor's approval. As some nutritional supplements may interact with certain medications and as they may adversely affect particular medical conditions, please consult your doctor before embarking on a course.

Part 1

1

What it means to have fibromyalgia

Fibromyalgia Syndrome (FMS for short) is a chronic condition of widespread pain. In addition to muscle, tendon, ligament and nerve pain, there is often heightened sensitivity of the skin and aching around the joints. *Fibro* means fibrous tissue i.e. tendons and ligaments, *my* means muscle, and *algia* means pain. The word Syndrome relates to a collection of symptoms that, when they occur together, identify an illness.

Symptoms

As well as persistent widespread pain, the symptoms commonly occurring with fibromyalgia include fatigue, difficulty sleeping, anxiety, irritable bowel syndrome, irritable bladder problems, depression, temperomandibular jaw (TMJ) dysfunction, headaches, anxiety, morning stiffness and 'brain fog' – difficulties with short-term memory and concentration. Some individuals are also troubled with thyroid problems, hypermobile joints, allergies, dermatological disorders, dizziness, sensitivity to light, dry eyes, and in women heavy periods, pelvic pain and painful sexual intercourse.

In fibromyalgia, several areas may hurt at one time, but one region in particular may be the cause of most concern. Also, the pain can seem to migrate from one area to another, for no reason that you can see. One day your neck may hurt so badly you can barely turn your head; the next, although your neck pain is mysteriously easing, your legs may ache so much that walking is difficult. If you can actually look back at your activities over the previous day or two, it's often possible to work out what caused the pain in a certain area. For instance, turning your head to speak to someone beside you for a couple of hours can cause pain in your neck and shoulder, and walking up a steep hill can make your legs and hips hurt.

Stress is one the greatest enemies of the fibromyalgia sufferer, as is the lack of restorative sleep, cold or humid weather conditions, too much activity or the wrong type of activity. Any one of these elements may provoke a 'flare-up' of symptoms – for example, muscle tightness and spasms, insomnia, disabling fatigue and heightened anxiety. A 'flare-up' can persist for days, weeks or even months.

The pain of fibromyalgia is just as individual to each person as fingerprints are. One person may experience searing, burning pains; another throbbing sensations; another tingling and numbness, another constant severe aching and another mild aches. When accompanied by a multitude of other symptoms and illnesses it is no wonder the individual can feel overwhelmed.

Until the last two decades or so, doctors believed their fibromyalgia patients to be psychosomatic – i.e. that their pain and other symptoms were prompted by mental factors such as internal conflict or stress. In other words, their symptoms were thought to be 'all in the mind'. Thankfully, that view is slowly changing and doctors are more aware of fibromyalgia as a solid medical condition.

Who gets fibromyalgia?

Approximately 80–90 per cent of fibromyalgia sufferers are women, and it normally appears during their childbearing years. However, men and children can also be affected – indeed, many adults with the condition believe they developed it in childhood. The average age at onset is 35–45 years, but it has been known to arise in adults over 70 years of age.

Fibromyalgia is very common, and it has been estimated that, world-wide, around ten per cent of the population is affected. As the symptoms of fibromyalgia vary so much in severity, some experts believe that many sufferers have either not yet consulted a doctor, or have had their health problems dismissed. Another reason for non-diagnosis is that many people fail to seek treatment because they are reluctant to admit that their body is not working as it should.

Research indicates that fibromyalgia can run in families. This may either be due to the family environment i.e. familial exposure to the same oil or gas fumes, aerosol sprays, glue, varnish etc., or it may be genetic in nature, being passed down through the generations. In some cases it can even be both. There is preliminary

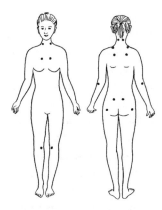

Figure 1.1 The 18 tender points used to establish a diagnosis of fibromyalgia

evidence suggesting that the condition can indeed be inherited, particularly by the female members in a family. Males have the same family genes, but their hormonal milieu appears to offer a measure of protection.

The diagnosis

People with fibromyalgia have areas of tenderness in specific locations – usually at junctions of muscle and bone. These areas are known as tender points and may be exquisitely painful when pressed. Otherwise they may or may not cause pain.

In 1990, the American College of Rheumatology defined the official criteria for the diagnosis of fibromyalgia. It is:

- pain in both sides of the body, pain above and below the waist, and pain along the spine, for more than three months;
- pain or tenderness in 11 out of 18 tender points, sited at specific locations in the body (see Figure 1.1).

The causes of fibromyalgia

Researchers have suggested that fibromyalgia is linked to the following:

- An imbalance in the chemical serotonin, which results in lowered pain tolerance and an unrestful sleep cycle. Low serotonin levels also cause the individual to be less physically active, and the muscles and other tissues to be more sensitive, painful and easily irritated. The resulting oversensitive nerve cells often leads to widespread soft tissue pain.

• An imbalance in the chemicals cortisol and growth hormone – the release of which is controlled by the pituitary gland and hypothalamus – causing fatigue, mood changes, poor concentration and short-term memory results. An imbalance can also cause a lowered tolerance to pain and other fibromyalgia symptoms.

• Disruption of 'delta-wave' sleep, which results in less growth hormone being manufactured by the body (growth hormone is largely produced during this deep phase of sleep). Disturbed sleep is believed to be both a cause and effect of fibromyalgia.

• Immune system disturbances resulting from an overload of environmental toxins – i.e. pesticides, aerosols, car fumes, food additives and preservatives etc.

Triggers for fibromyalgia

The above dysfunctions can be triggered by the following:

• a viral illness such as the 'flu or glandular fever;
• a neck injury (whiplash injuries are thought to be the chief trigger of fibromyalgia);
• surgery;
• emotional trauma and stress.

A dietary answer

Fibromyalgia is a disease in which the balance of the body is affected. There are problems within the immune system (our antibody protection against disease), the endocrine system (our hormone levels) and the central nervous system (our body's nerve signalling system located in the brain and spinal cord). These systems need to be supported by working from every angle possible to help the body back into balance. When, as a result, the bodily systems are once again networking properly, the errors will begin to correct themselves. The most vital area of support is improved nutrition, for among its many benefits, it is of enormous help to the body at the important cellular level.

2

Basic considerations for health

Hunger is the body's alarm system telling us to eat. When our blood sugar levels are low, the body sends out this alarm, telling us to eat sugars, and when the body needs more liquid, it sends out an alarm telling us to drink. However, few people recognize that the body sends out alarms when a diet is lacking something it needs. These alarms come in the form of lethargy, sleeplessness, low mood, miscellaneous aches and pains and, eventually, chronic disease. It makes sense, then, to say that healing can best come from improvements in nutrition.

You may be surprised to hear that food is one of the finest medicines we can put into our bodies, that it is one of the best means of influencing our health – but it is true. Not only does food keep us alive, it also has the ability to repair and regenerate our body's tissues.

Unfortunately, however, our diets have become very poor over the years. Nowadays, because of chemical pesticides, food additives, preservatives and so on, we constantly ingest low levels of toxins, which has given rise to an array of immune disorders. Fibromyalgia is one such disorder.

Why good nutrition?

The human body possesses all the necessary systems for regeneration, rejuvenation and repair. When provided with the right conditions, mentally and physically, the body will quite often heal itself, working at optimum efficiency and staving off disease. The most important factor influencing good physical health is good nutrition. This is because it allows our cells – the smallest but most important components in our bodies – to be nourished continually and washed clean of waste. The cells will not function efficiently if they are seldom fed and cleansed.

Poor nutrition, on the other hand, causes a gradual toxic build-up within the cells. It can even lead to cell death. 'Junk food' is a fine example of poor nutrition, for not only does it carry few nutrients, its digestion and detoxification draws energy from the body that could otherwise be used in thinking, working, playing and so on. In addition, poor-quality foods are difficult for the body to eliminate. As a result, bowel movements become irregular and toxic substances are absorbed into the body.

Many experts believe that fibromyalgia may arise as a result of toxic overload. When the liver – our main detoxification organ – is unable to keep up with the removal of toxins, they are deposited in the muscle fibres and connective tissues, causing pain and discomfort.

As you can see, then, it is vital that people with fibromyalgia eat the right foods. Disease occurs when the body is vulnerable, when it is run down and crying out for help – shown by fatigue, anxiety, insomnia, low mood and so on. However, when the cause of the problem is being treated, rather than the effect – as is the case when a nutritious diet is being followed – healing is likely to take place.

In fibromyalgia, there are abnormalities in the immune system (antibody protection against disease), the endocrine system (hormone levels) and the central nervous system (the body's nerve signalling system located in the brain and spinal cord). This book is dedicated to suggesting the foods and nutritional supplements you can use to help return these systems to normal.

The way we were

Our bodies, physiologically speaking, have barely changed since the Stone Age. Available foodstuffs remain largely unchanged, too. What has changed, and in a relatively short period of time, is our diet and behaviour. We now eat a wide variety of 'processed' foods – that is, foods grown using chemicals and preservatives, flavourings, colourings and so on added before we eat them – in a stressful environment.

Stone Age people, on the other hand, had all the time in the world, except when under direct threat. Their foods were not sprayed with chemicals or injected with preservatives, they were eaten fresh and in season – and fresh, uncontaminated fruit and vegetables are highly nutritious. They are also rich in 'enzymes' – the substances that aid digestion. For the most part, the food was uncooked, too. Unfortunately, cooking above 41°C (107°F) and refrigeration both destroy the live digestive enzymes that help our bodies to break down food.

Stone Age people would also have eaten one type of food at a time. For example, when blackberries came into season, they would make whole meals of this fruit. This is quite unlike what we do today, when we combine several types of food at one sitting. It is a sad fact that we generally place more importance on taste than quality.

Fed on freshly gathered, uncontaminated foods, the digestive systems of Stone Age people would have functioned superbly, and the added benefit of fresh air and exercise contributed to their good health. It is doubtful that Stone Age people developed fibromyalgia. This disorder has seemingly become prevalent only in the last 100 years and, unfortunately, its incidence is rising all the time.

Foodstuffs today

Since our Stone Age ancestors, we have developed the following habits so that, in modern times:

- we eat food grown on artificially fertilized land and sprayed several times with chemical pesticides (poisons), which kill essential soil microbes that would otherwise help plants to absorb the nutrient-rich minerals essential to good health;
- plant foods are then artificially ripened, stored and processed;
- we generally prefer taste to quality;
- we eat foods out of season because they are readily available;
- we eat the tasty parts of the food only, disposing of the rest – for example, wheat husks are removed before the remaining cereal is processed into white flour – but 'whole' foods aid the removal of waste materials from the bowel, so are vital to good bowel health;
- we eat hurriedly, often while working or thinking about problems;
- we dilute the nutrients in our food by drinking at the same time.

Food sensitivities and fibromyalgia

It has been well remarked that food sensitivities and fibromyalgia go hand in hand. In a survey published in the journal *Clinical Rheumatology*, 42 per cent of people with fibromyalgia said their symptoms worsened after eating certain foods. The study at the University of Oslo, Norway, found that nearly a quarter of people with the condition had tried diet therapy, with 46 per cent reporting less pain and stiffness, and 36 per cent reduced joint swelling. The types of offending foods do vary. Some people find they are sensitive to gluten, others to dairy products, while still others might not be able to tolerate soy, corn, some preservatives, or sweeteners such as aspartame and MSG. In other words, the offending food varies widely from individual to individual, and what works for one person may not work for another. Some doctors say this is because fibro-myalgia is a symptom complex or umbrella condition, rather than a specific illness, with different mechanisms and causes, and with different conditions responding to different nutritional approaches. Conditions sometimes associated with fibromyalgia include migraine, chronic pain including myofascial pain syndrome (referred pain from 'trigger points' or knots of constantly contracted muscles), diabetes, sleep apnoea and Sjögren's syndrome (dry eyes and mouth).

In some cases, the different responses to foods are believed to be linked with another underlying, maybe undiagnosed illness. For example, thyroid disease, vitamin D deficiency (see page 36) and coeliac disease are all differential diagnoses where the individual's food response may be significant. Giving up wheat products such as bread, cake and pastries, for example, will improve wellbeing for people with gluten intolerance or sensitivity. People with hypothy-roidism (sluggish thyroid) should go easy on raw brassicas (cabbage, Brussels sprouts, broccoli and cauliflower), as they contain goitro-gens, chemicals that interfere with thyroid hormone function.

A diet low in purines is usually recommended for gout, so reducing consumption of red meat, poultry and fish may help such individuals. Restless legs syndrome might respond well to an increase in iron-rich foods and perhaps a supplement.

It may also be that food sensitivities themselves can account for symptoms such as discomfort and tiredness. Take a careful note of which foods you respond to, as this may be a pointer to any under-lying health problems.

Gluten

Some research has found a strong association between gluten intol-erance and fibromyalgia. A 2013 Spanish study found a 'remarkable prevalence' of coeliac disease in people with both irritable bowel syndrome and fibromyalgia, in comparison to those who had just irritable bowel syndrome alone. At the Central University Hospital of Asturias (HUCA), Professor Luis Rodrigo and colleagues postulated that some cases of fibromyalgia could actually be undiagnosed coeliac disease. The research suggested that in some individuals, gluten may trigger auto-immune inflammation in the digestive tract which in turn might set off or exacerbate FMS, in line with the triad of IBS, chronic fatigue and muscle pain noted by other research, and it is speculated that there might be a common underlying food sensitivity.

Oxalates

The theory that fibromyalgia might be linked to oxalates was personally tested by Dr Clare Morrison, a GP writing in the Daily Mail in 2012. Dr Morrison said her own debilitating fibromyalgia symptoms vanished when she cut out foods rich in oxalates – natural compounds found in 'healthy' foods such as fruit, vegetables, salad, nuts and beans. 'More in desperation than expectation, I tried a low-oxalate diet, cutting out virtually all 'healthy' food – I avoided most fruits and vegetables, salads, beans, nuts, wheatgerm, soya — as well as tea, coffee and chocolate,' says Dr Morrison (*Daily Mail*, July and August 2012).

Oxalates are a kind of inbuilt pesticide in many plants – nature's way of deterring predators such as insects. It is well-documented that if sheep and cattle eat large quantities of high-oxalate plants, they can develop problems such as staggering, stiffness, weakness and even kidney failure. In humans, the theory is that in certain individuals, oxalates may accumulate in the muscles, brain and urinary system if not excreted properly, especially if they are low on calcium, as calcium binds with oxalate in the bowel, preventing it from being absorbed.

A low-oxalate diet means avoiding certain fruits and vegetables which are high in oxalates, such as berries (blueberries, blackberries, etc.), oranges, rhubarb, beetroot, celery, spinach, potatoes, leeks, carrots, green peppers and parsnips. Beans are also not recommended, including baked beans, kidney beans and green beans. You also need to cut out tea, coffee, chocolate, cocoa, nuts, soya and wheatgerm (bran cereals, wholemeal bread).

For a full list of low- and high-oxalate foods, see <ohf.org/docs/Oxalate2008.pdf>.

Recommendations for fibromyalgia

In order to begin healing itself, the body requires a wide variety of foods and food combinations. To eat the same foods repeatedly means missing out on many important building blocks of life, for certain foods build and regenerate only certain parts of the body. A restricted diet also increases the risk of developing immune system disorders such as fibromyalgia.

Because the majority of our foodstuffs are grown in a chemical environment, they are low in nutrients and high in toxicity. It is advisable, therefore, to purchase organically grown produce and look for foods that are without added chemicals (colourings, flavourings, preservatives and so on).

Essential guidelines for achieving healing from fibromyalgia are as follows.

- Eat three or four small meals a day, with snacks in between.
- Never go more than two to three hours without eating, which means you should never go hungry.
- Do not skip breakfast. After fasting during the night, the body needs glucose. When nourishment is withheld, brain function is diminished. Studies have shown that children who eat breakfast perform better at school than those who have not eaten.
- Avoid missing a meal. When we allow ourselves to become very hungry, the sugary, high-fat foods that are bad for us become more tempting.
- Ensure your snacks are nutritious and readily available. Good examples are raw fruits and vegetables, fruit and vegetable juices, dried fruit, unsalted uncoated nuts (unless you have a nut allergy, of course), a variety of seeds and rye crispbreads. These should not spoil your appetite for an upcoming meal. At least 40 per cent of your calorie intake should be made up of 'complex' carbohydrates. These include fruits, vegetables and whole grains, such as bulgar wheat, couscous, millet, barley, brown rice and whole wheat (see Chapter 3 for more information).
- Lightly steam your vegetables. Over-cooking them removes much of their nutritious content.
- Make meals that can be frozen in individual servings.
- Fats (oils) should comprise approximately 30 per cent of your calorie intake. Unsaturated fats (also known as polyunsaturated

fats) are greatly beneficial to health. These include olive, safflower, sunflower and corn oils. Saturated fats, however, are largely derived from animals and should be consumed in moderation, if at all. Examples are lard, suet, butter and dripping (see Chapter 3 for more information).

- Protein should make up approximately 30 per cent of your total calorie intake. Sources include chicken, turkey, fish (including tuna and salmon), beans, legumes (peas, beans and peanuts). Red meat is considered by some experts to be detrimental to fibromyalgics. However, my opinion is that small cuts of lean red meat, eaten only once or twice a week, are harmless. Meat is also one of the few sources of vitamin B12 (see Chapter 3 for more information on protein).
- Eat plenty of fibre in the form of fruits, vegetables, wholegrain breads, cereals and legumes (see Chapter 3 for more information).
- Minimize your intake of sugar. Use raw honey, date sugar, molasses, barley malt and so on in place of table sugar and artificial sweeteners, such as aspartame and saccharin (see Chapter 6 for more information on sugar and aspartame).
- Junk foods and fast foods are loaded with harmful additives. Avoid them if at all possible.
- Look out for additives on food labels. Flavourings, colourings and preservatives are often presented as 'E' numbers.
- Avoid refined and processed foods. Those that come in tins, jars and packets almost certainly contain additives (except for most foods purchased in healthfood shops). Fresh foods, on the other hand, are usually additive-free.
- Try to avoid caffeine, chocolate, cola drinks, alcohol and smoking. They may be enjoyable, but are especially detrimental in fibromyalgia (see Chapter 6 for more information on 'stimulants').
- Avoid drinking for at least half an hour before and half an hour after eating. Liquid dilutes the nutritional value of our food.
- Due to the high fibre content of the fibromyalgia healing diet, try to drink eight to ten glasses of water a day, inclusive of fruit/vegetable juices and herbal teas. Distilled or filtered water is highly recommended (see Chapter 7 for more information). Mineral water is not recommended as it is not very effective in drawing mineral salts and other debris out of the tissues.

However, if there is nothing other than water straight from the tap, mineral water is the better choice.

- Ensure you are not consuming large quantities of salt. Remember that it is commonly used as a preservative and added to most processed, prepackaged foods anyway. I recommend that you use minimal amounts in cooking and at the table. Rock salt, sea salt and 'Bioforce' seasonings are healthier alternatives, but should still be used sparingly (the latter are available from healthfood shops or the address given in the Useful addresses section at the back of the book).
- Only take medication when you really need to. This will reduce the number of unnecessary toxins entering your body.
- Take the recommended vitamin and mineral supplements. Because people with fibromyalgia suffer many nutritional deficiencies, supplements – tablet-form concentrates of a particular vitamin, mineral and so on – are essential. Some nutritional supplements are required in high doses for a few months, after which a small maintenance dose should be taken (more about supplements for fibromyalgia in Chapter 5).
- Take antioxidant supplements to protect the cells and help release energy (see the Useful addresses section at the back of this book for recommended suppliers of antioxidants and other supplements, and Chapter 5 for more information about antioxidants).

This book describes the recommended day-to-day diet for people with fibromyalgia, including the supplements known to be useful in treating the condition. It also outlines, in Chapter 7, a 21-day detoxification programme that will help the body to eliminate stored toxins and debris. I advise, however, that you gradually accustom yourself to the new foods in this diet; that you get used to eating cleanly grown produce and additive-free foods for at least a month prior to embarking on the detoxification programme. This will give your body, and tastebuds, time to adjust to the changes to your diet and minimize any possible side-effects arising from detoxification (more about these in Chapter 7).

Osteoporosis and fibromyalgia

The reduced activity levels common in people with fibromyalgia can lead to the early onset of osteoporosis, where the bones become brittle and more prone to fracturing. If left untreated, the condition can painlessly progress until a fracture occurs. Any bone can be fractured, but fractures of the spine and hip are of most concern due to their risk of serious consequences.

The condition is four times more common in women than in men, and a woman is more vulnerable if she is post-menopausal and experienced an early menopause. Unfortunately, I developed osteoporosis before I began to alter my diet, and it's not so easy to reverse. If you think you're at risk of this disease, ask your doctor to refer you to your local hospital for a bone density scan.

If you are diagnosed with osteoporosis, you will be prescribed medication to help your bones retain their calcium. Eating a calcium-rich diet can also prevent further calcium loss. Calcium-containing foods include dairy produce, dark green leafy vegetables (such as spinach, broccoli, spring cabbage and Brussels sprouts), shrimp, canned salmon and sardines, black strap molasses, calcium-fortified low-fat tofu and almonds. Some commercial foods, such as certain orange juices, cereals and yogurts are fortified with calcium, and are highly recommended. It's advisable that, even if you have fibromyalgia and are not diagnosed with osteoporosis, you eat a diet that is rich in calcium and vitamin D (see page 36). Such a diet will help to prevent the future development of this bone-thinning disease. Drinking milk fortified with vitamin D is another good option – vitamin D is vital for enabling digested calcium to enter the bones.

You should also be aware that fresh fruits and vegetables contain essential minerals such as magnesium and potassium which help to reduce the elimination of calcium from the body. Magnesium-rich foods include dairy products, potatoes, beetroot, nuts, spinach, sole and halibut. Potassium-rich foods include bananas, oranges, prunes, potatoes, carrots, broccoli, avocados, lima beans, mushrooms, celery, alfalfa and cantaloupes. It's also worth noting that skimmed milk and non-fat dairy products provide as much calcium as full-fat milk and dairy products.

Recent research has shown that individuals who include more unsaturated fat in their diet (see 'Fats and lipids' in Chapter 3) are, on average, better able to absorb calcium than those on a low-fat diet. Therefore, the diet in this book advocates that 30 per cent of your food intake is fat in the form of polyunsaturated oils (canola, sunflower, olive and so on), as well as oily fish, avocados, nuts and seeds.

3

Necessary foods

The foods necessary for the treatment of fibromyalgia include:

- protein
- carbohydrate
- fat
- fibre.

The average diet in the West is composed of 60–70 per cent carbohydrates, 5–10 per cent protein and 25–45 per cent fat (most of it saturated, not unsaturated – see pages 22–3). These figures are based on percentages of calories, not grams. Eating such proportions of the different food groups invariably results in loss of muscle tone and shape, swings in energy and endurance, and slower mental focus (including concentration and short-term memory). As these problems are usually present anyway in fibromyalgia, it makes sense to say that improving your diet can greatly reduce the symptoms.

Studies of people with fibromyalgia have also shown that they lack the following:

- one of the important building blocks of life i.e. the constituent that repairs muscle;
- an important transition fuel that helps to break down fat;
- a particular fuel source that results in reactive hypoglycaemia – a deficiency of glucose in the bloodstream.

The basic components of muscle and other soft tissues are proteins and minerals. Research has shown, though, that the average fibromyalgia sufferer eats a diet that is high in carbohydrates and low in protein – that was certainly me before I became interested in diet as a treatment. The human body is capable of repairing muscle and other soft tissues, but when it's deficient in protein, this restorative process will not take place. In fact, a diet low in protein will lead to increased pain.

So what can you actually eat? The diet recommended for the treatment of fibromyalgia comprises of 40 per cent *carbohydrate*, 30 per cent *protein* and 30 per cent *unsaturated fat*. These essential nutrients provide our bodies with vital energy and, as our bodies are in a constant state of regeneration, serve as fundamental building materials. You should also try to eat a moderately high amount of fibre (see page 24). *Vitamins* and *minerals* are of almost equal importance and will be discussed in Chapter 5.

It may not surprise you to know that junk or fast food is not recommended for people with fibromyalgia – or for healthy people for that matter. Individuals can survive on junk food for a while because it is comprised mainly of carbohydrates and fat, which have a high energy value. However, because junk food is short of sustaining nutrients, the body will not continue to repair and regenerate indefinitely. It slowly becomes clogged up and lethargic, like a cog wheel that is fed treacle instead of oil.

Our bodies also need a regular input of enzymes to function at optimum levels. As mentioned earlier, enzymes are crucial to good digestion and many of them are provided by fresh raw food. Enzymes speed up the chemical reactions within our bodies and are essential to good health. Without sufficient enzymes, we deprive ourselves of the necessary nutrients. It is important to know that enzymes are easily destroyed in cooking and processing, so it is advisable to eat two to four portions of raw fruit and/or vegetables each day.

In total, we should try to consume five portions of fruit and five portions of vegetables a day, as recommended by the World Health Organization. Each of the following is equivalent to one portion:

- 100 g (4 oz) of a very large fruit, such as watermelon, melon or pineapple;
- a large fruit, such as an orange, banana or apple;
- 2 medium fruits, such as kiwi fruit, plums or satsumas;
- 100 ml (3 fl oz) freshly squeezed fruit or vegetable juice;
- 100 g (4 oz) berries or cherries;
- a large bowl of salad;
- 90 g (3½ oz) – cooked weight – green vegetables;
- 75 g (3 oz) – cooked weight – root vegetables, such as carrot or swede, but do not include potatoes, sweet potatoes or yams;

- 75 g (3 oz) – cooked weight – small vegetables, such as peas or sweetcorn;
- 75 g (3 oz) pulses.

Of equal importance is that our diets contain sufficient roughage. This fibrous and bulking content of foods reduces the transit time of substances within the bowel. However, roughage is lost in food that has been refined. Thus, instead of being rapidly eliminated, refined food can sit in the bowel for much longer than it should, the resulting toxicity being reabsorbed into the body as it putrefies and rots there.

Protein

As our bodies are constructed of protein, a good, steady supply is essential. Protein is vital to tissue regeneration and maintenance. It is also largely responsible for the production of hormones and the cells involved in immunity.

Digestive enzymes are required for protein synthesis, the transforming of proteins into repair constituents, which are used for cell regeneration. We need 22 amino acids, 14 of which can be produced by the body. The remaining 8 must be supplied by our food. All 22 amino acids are required at the same time and in the right quantity for protein synthesis. If just one is in short supply, the production of protein will be much reduced. It may even cease altogether. We have, therefore, a vital rationale for the consumption of sufficient protein-containing foods. (More about amino acids and enzymes later.)

It may surprise you to know that a vegetarian diet that does not contain sufficient grain can cause protein foods to synthesize to form *carbohydrate* instead of protein – any excess carbohydrate being converted to fat. However, animal protein – meat, chicken, fish, dairy produce and eggs – contains all the essential amino acids and is one of the very few sources of vitamin B12. Unfortunately, animal protein contains no fibre – an essential ingredient of the fibromyalgia healing diet. Instead, it can be loaded with saturated fat and cholesterol, which have a negative effect on the body. For these reasons, the fibromyalgia healing diet specifies only a small amount of animal protein. Dairy products should be consumed in moderation, too.

Fibromyalgia-friendly sources of protein are lean red meat, poultry, fish, tuna, soya products (all of which should be served in reasonably small helpings), cottage cheese, seeds, nuts and legumes. In a week, a serving of meat or fish no larger than the palm of your hand should be eaten on two to three occasions, and two to three organic, free-range eggs should be consumed. If you can find omega 3-fortified eggs, all the better – it may say on the box 'fed with DHA and EHA'. Butter should be spread very thinly on your wholegrain bread and rye crispbreads. In place of cows' milk, use soya milk, which is rich in protein, or rice milk, which has a high carbohydrate content. Goats' milk is an acceptable alternative, too. (There is further information on soya products towards the end of this chapter.)

Although vegetables and fruits are rich in fibre, carbohydrate and certain vitamins and minerals, they are low in protein. Nuts and legumes are excellent sources of protein, but must be combined to achieve a full range of amino acids, for example brown rice and lentils. However, a diet comprised mainly of nuts and legumes would render the individual vitamin B12 deficient.

It is a fact that people who eat a lot of grain products – bread, pasta, rice, cereals and so on – in an effort to limit their fat intake are likely to be consuming insufficient protein. This can lead to weakening of the immune system, which is suppressed in fibromyalgia anyway. If protein intake is low, the body will pull protein from the muscles, which then has the effect of slowing down the metabolism (the rate of conversion of food to energy). Protein deficiency causes low energy, low stamina, weakness, poor resistance to infection, depression and slow healing of wounds.

The consequences of a high-protein diet being uncertain, an interesting study into the effects of different quantities of protein intake was conducted in 2000.[1] It showed, surprisingly, that a high-protein diet can improve antioxidant status (read how important antioxidants are in Chapter 4). However, it is now commonly known that a very high intake of protein may cause the tissues to be overly acidic, which can promote degenerative disease. Protein deficiency, on the other hand, causes oxidative stress, with the result that the immune system is weakened and inflammatory disorders of the arthritic type are likely to arise. I would advise, therefore, that approximately 20–25 per cent of your total daily calories consist of protein.

Please do not worry too much about percentages, however. If you at least try to consume the recommended amounts of meat, as well as fruit, vegetables, nuts, seeds, legumes, soft-boiled egg yolks, soya products and so on – the suggested menus in Chapter 7 may give you a better idea of quantities – you will be doing your body a great favour. Remember, too, that healing changes will come about even if you are not able to follow this diet to the letter. Simply do the best you can and appreciate the fact that you are helping your body to fight this disease.

Although I do not advocate counting calories in the fibromyalgia healing diet, the following calorific values should give you a rough idea of not only your protein intake but also of your total calorific consumption (examples of carbohydrate and fat calories are given later in this chapter). Depending on your levels of activity – you are not likely to be very active if you are in a lot of pain – you should be eating between 1800 and 3000 calories a day.

Here are the calorific contents of some common protein foods:

- 28 g (1 oz) grilled haddock – a very small piece – provides 40 calories;
- 28 g (1 oz) roasted chicken – also a very small piece – provides 40 calories;
- 28 g (1 oz) cottage cheese provides 15 calories;
- 28 g (1 oz) Parmesan cheese provides 120 calories;
- 28 g (1 oz) soya beans provides 50 calories;
- 28 g (1 oz) butter provides 226 calories – so, to reiterate, butter should be used very sparingly.

Soya products

The reduced activity levels common in people with fibromyalgia can lead to the early onset of osteoporosis. This is particularly likely among postmenopausal women. However, soya foods are believed to contain plant oestrogens – oestrogen being one of the hormones that are in short supply during and after the meno-pause as mentioned earlier. These have the effect of preventing bone density loss and reducing hot flushes, irritability, aching joints and depression – all of which are symptoms of the meno-pause. During a study in 2000, Japanese researchers concluded that the postmenopausal women who had consumed the highest amounts of soya-containing foods – such as tofu, soya milk and boiled soya beans – had increased bone mass and fewer backaches

11/4

EVANS

4/11

Euros

and aching joints than those who had consumed less of such foods.[2]

I would like to add a word of warning, however. Although rich in protein and very nutritious, high levels of soya consumption can suppress thyroid function. Because soya acts as a hormone in the body, it can interact with the delicate balance of thyroxine – the hormone produced by the thyroid gland. Consuming large amounts of soya products is capable of disrupting the thyroid gland, causing hypothyroidism (the state where thyroid levels are consistently too low). Pre-existing hypothyroidism may also be worsened.

My advice is, then, to drink no more than one glass of soya milk a day, maybe substituting a glass of rice milk later on. Other soya products, such as tofu, boiled soya beans and textured soya meats (sometimes called textured vegetable proteins – TVP) should be eaten on not more than one occasion every alternate day.

Carbohydrate

Carbohydrates – foods such as fruits, vegetables and grains (wholemeal bread, pasta, brown rice, cereals, couscous, millet, barley, bulgar wheat and other cereals) – supply our bodies with energy. Our digestive systems break down carbohydrates into simple sugars that are used to fuel essential body processes, such as brain function, nervous system function and muscle activity – all of which are problem areas in fibromyalgia. Any excess carbohydrate is converted to fat by insulin, the 'fat-storage' hormone.

To guarantee the production of sufficient energy and ensure that fats and proteins are effectively broken down, we need to eat plenty of 'complex' carbohydrates. These include fruits, vegetables, whole-grain breads, wholemeal pastas, brown rice, potatoes and sweetcorn. 'Simple' carbohydrates are the sugars found in table sugar, sweets, cakes and sweetened cereals. They provide a spurt of energy, but, in the long term, can cause blood sugar levels to fluctuate erratically. Simple carbohydrates should, therefore, be avoided as much as possible.

I reiterate that we should all try to eat five portions of fruit and five portions of vegetables a day, remembering that raw vegetables offer greater nutritional value than those that have been cooked. Organically grown fruit and vegetables are highly recommended – 'organic' meaning grown without the presence of chemical pesticides and other toxins. Cleanly grown produce can now be found on our supermarket shelves and it is generally not much higher in price than chemically treated and grown foods.

As approximately half of our calorie intake should consist of carbohydrates, the calorific values of some recommended sources are as follows:

- 28 g (1 oz) banana provides 22 calories;
- 28 g (1 oz) orange provides 12 calories;
- 28 g (1 oz) apple provides 17 calories;
- 28 g (1 oz) wholemeal pasta provides 35 calories;
- 28 g (1 oz) wholemeal (also called wholegrain) bread provides 38 calories;
- 28 g (1 oz) cauliflower provides 3 calories;
- 28 g (1 oz) cabbage provides 4 calories.

Fats and lipids (oils)

Unfortunately, it is a fallacy that the answer to losing weight is simply to cut down on fat. Fats (fatty acids) are the most concentrated sources of energy in our diet –1 g fat providing the body with 9 calories of energy. Fat-containing foods are crucial to health as they slow the absorption of carbohydrates into the bloodstream, thus limiting the production of insulin, which is essential for controlling blood sugar levels. (Glucose, or blood sugar, is one of our body's most important nutrients and the basic source of energy for mind and body.)

There are two types of fats.

- **Saturated fats** These come mainly from animal sources and are generally solid at room temperature. For many years, margarine was believed to be a healthier choice than butter. However, it is now known that some of the fats in the hydrogenation process involved in making margarine are changed into 'trans-fatty acids' and the body metabolizes these as if they were saturated fatty acids – the same as butter. Although butter should be used very sparingly, it is also a valuable source of oils and vitamin A. Margarine, on the other hand, is an artificial product containing many additives.

- **Unsaturated fats** are often called 'polyunsaturated' or 'mono-unsaturated' fats. These types of fats are derived mainly from vegetables, nuts and seeds, and are usually liquid at room temperature. Examples of unsaturated fats are olive, rapeseed, safflower and sunflower oils.

While saturated fats are believed to be implicated in the development of heart disease, unsaturated fats actually have a protective effect. These omega 3 and omega 6 fatty acids are obtained from vegetable oils, seeds (sunflower seeds, sesame seeds, linseeds and so on), nuts, avocados and oily fish (mackerel, herring, tuna and others).

Olive oil is considered the superior source of these acids as it suffers less damage during cooking than other oils. All oils should be stored in sealed containers in a cool, dark place to prevent the onset of rancidity.

A fatty acid not often mentioned is omega 9, but if you suffer from inflammation it's just as important. It's often said that fibromyalgia is not an inflammatory condition, but in my worst years my neck and back were severely inflamed, and my wrists were so painful and swollen I was unable to move them and wore wrist braces all the time. It's clear, then, that fibromyalgia can cause inflammation, which can be reduced or eliminated by regular intake of omega 9 fatty acid. This acid is present in sesame and olive oil, avocados, peanuts, macadamia nuts, cashews, pistachios and pecans.

Oils are a natural source of vitamin E, which is an important antioxidant. Antioxidants are essential to cell life because they mop up destructive 'free radicals' within the body (see Chapter 5 for more information about antioxidants and free radicals). Unfortunately, during processing, the vitamin E in some unsaturated oils is removed, depriving the body of this vitamin. Processed oils are also very susceptible to rancidity. It is recommended, therefore, that you obtain your fats from natural sources (see above), including cold-pressed vegetable oils.

It is important to note that the process of frying changes the molecular structure of foods, rendering them potentially damaging to the body. If you must fry something, it is best to use a small amount of extra virgin olive oil and cook at a low temperature.

Sautéing in a little water or tomato juice can be quite acceptable, but, otherwise, grilling, baking and steaming are great alternatives. A word of warning – never reheat used oils, for this, too, can be harmful to the body.

You've probably heard that eggs are high in cholesterol, and that therefore they are harmful to health. However, cholesterol is an important constituent of cell membranes, and we've already heard that good cell health is vital. It's only when large amounts of cholesterol are consumed that plaques of fatty material can be deposited on the artery walls – a condition called atherosclerosis. Eggs are also known to contain lecithin, which is a superb biological 'detergent' that is capable of breaking down fats so they can be used by the body. Eggs should be soft-boiled or poached, as a hard yolk will bind the lecithin, rendering it useless as a 'fat detergent'. Although I have recommended that you eat two to three eggs a week, those following the fibromyalgia healing diet on a vegetarian basis should eat up to five eggs a week to obtain the necessary protein. More than five can cause cholesterol levels to be too high.

It is estimated that the fat intake of most adults is 42 per cent of their total daily calories, and that this figure mostly consists of saturated fat. In fibromyalgia, the recommended daily intake is 30 per cent, i.e. just over 28 grams (1 oz). This equates to only 320 calories. Eating the necessary unsaturated fat will ensure reduced calorie intake and greater energy provision.

Here are the calorific values of some fat-containing foods:

- 28 g (1 oz) oil contains 130 calories;
- 28 g (1 oz) butter contains 226 calories;
- 28 g (1 oz) eggs contains 80 calories;
- 28 g (1 oz) oily fish contains 60 calories.

Fibre (roughage)

A type of carbohydrate, fibre is the indigestible parts of plants. It is the cellulose fibres forming the leaf webbing in green vegetables, it is the skins of sweetcorn and beans, and it is the husks of wheat and corn. Foods containing fibre include fruits, vegetables, nuts, seeds, beans, peas, lentils, wholemeal breads and cereals (wheat, oats, rye, barley, corn and so on). In fact, a large percentage of the foods recommended in the fibromyalgia healing diet contain fibre, and the above-mentioned are all highly nutritious foods, providing not only fibre but also starch and many essential vitamins and minerals. You may have heard of the highly successful 'F-Plan Diet'. One of the most compelling reasons that fibre became popular in weight-loss programmes was because the appetite is satiated on far fewer calories. This important food constituent also ensures slower and more regulated absorption of glucose into the bloodstream. As a result, you avoid plummeting into hunger troughs and craving sugars to raise blood sugar levels. However, please note that a very high-fibre diet can impede the absorption of essential vitamins and minerals. It is important, therefore, that you don't vastly overdo the fibre.

Nutritionists have labelled fibre 'nature's broom' because it quickly sweeps the system clean, ensuring no unhealthy waste products lurk in hidden corners. When waste persistently lingers in the bowel, as happens in low-fibre diets, immune system disorders often result. Fibromyalgia is one such disorder.

A moderately high fibre intake will, therefore, speed up the transit time of material in the large bowel, limiting the amount of toxins absorbed back into the bloodstream from the digestive tract. As toxicity and irritable bowel syndrome (characterized by alternating bouts of constipation and diarrhoea) are both linked to fibromyalgia, I recommend that each meal has some fibre content. Furthermore, because of the bulking capacity of fibre, high levels of water consumption are necessary. I recommend, therefore, that eight to ten glasses of water – including the liquid in fruit/vegetable drinks and herbal teas – should be drunk daily. The water in coffee and tea (even decaffeinated), caffeinated soft drinks and alcohol does not count. Drinks containing caffeine are diuretics and actually make the body *lose* fluid. Alcohol can lead to dehydration, too.

Salt

Although our bodies need the sodium we obtain from salt, high intakes of it have a detrimental effect in many ways. High blood pressure and heart disease are only two conditions that are commonly linked to diets high in salt. A food 'additive', salt is used in virtually all processed foods as a preservative as it has the capacity to inhibit the growth of harmful micro-organisms. It is also added in large amounts to most breakfast cereals, except for shredded wheat products and a few others.

I would recommend that small amounts of sea or rock salt be used in baking, that a small amount of this mineral-rich salt be added to cooking, but that you try to avoid sprinkling any type of salt over your meals. Gradually reducing your intake of salt is the best way to retrain your palate.

The only exception to this rule is that people in hot climates and those who sweat a lot should ensure that lost salt is always replaced, as sweating causes sodium levels to drop.

4

Why diet is important in treating fibromyalgia

People with fibromyalgia suffer from the following:

- suppressed immune systems;
- the processing of nerve sensations is confused;
- certain hormone levels are abnormal;
- the soft tissues (muscles, tendons and ligaments) are low in energy and clogged with waste materials.

There is, undoubtedly, a lot to be corrected! We will see, in this chapter, how an improved diet can address some of the underlying causes of fibromyalgia.

Amino acids

The components that affect all of the above-mentioned systems and processes are amino acids, which are known as 'the building blocks of life'. Their functions include cell manufacture, muscle and tissue repair and the manufacture of antibodies. A total of 22 amino acids are capable of being produced when protein is broken down by the digestive process, 8 of these being essential because they cannot be manufactured by the body. With proper nutrition, the remaining 14 can be manufactured, however.

Although no studies have, as yet, been conducted in this respect, some experts are of the opinion that a certain branch chain of amino acids holds the key to the cause and treatment of fibromyalgia. The chain in question includes amino acids called 'tryptophan' and 'tyrosine', both of which are transported through the gut by the same protein molecule. People with fibromyalgia are known to have reduced levels of these two amino acids. In fact, tryptophan and tyrosine are now known to be especially susceptible to damage by toxicity and, as mentioned earlier, it is becoming increasingly evident that fibromyalgia can arise as a result of toxicity problems.

Below is a description of the affected amino acids, together with a corrective treatment.

- **Tryptophan** Tryptophan produces serotonin – a calming, pain-reducing chemical substance that is known to be deficient in fibromyalgia. Tryptophan-rich foods include fish, turkey, chicken, avocados, bananas, cottage cheese and wheatgerm. However, when the tryptophan carrier molecule is damaged, as is believed to be the case in fibromyalgia, the aforementioned foods may not be converted into serotonin. 5-Hydroxytryptophan (5-HTP), though, is capable of successfully raising serotonin levels. This enzyme, which is available as a supplement from specialist suppliers and healthfood shops, does not have the side-effects that often arise with pharmaceutical serotonin-enhancing medications, so it can be a valuable alternative to them. The recommended daily dose for fibromyalgics is 100–500 mg, depending on the severity of symptoms. It should be taken an hour before bedtime with a carbohydrate food, such as wholemeal toast, rice or oat cakes, rye crispbread and so on, to encourage improved sleep. I would, however, strongly advise that you consult your doctor before taking this supplement.
- **Tyrosine** This important amino acid is the precursor to the thyroid hormones. It is involved in the transmission of nerve impulses to the brain; improving memory; increasing mental alertness and promoting healthy functioning of the thyroid gland. Long-term improvements in the symptoms of fibromyalgia have been seen as a result of electro-acupuncture, which works in exactly the same way as conventional acupuncture, with the exception that electrical stimulation is used in place of needles. A TENS (Transcutaneous Electrical Nerve Stimulation) machine with surface electrodes, used for 30 minutes twice to seven times a week, can also be effective. Your local physiotherapy department may be able to provide further information.

We have known for several years that stress and/or physical trauma from, for example, a traffic accident or surgery, can trigger fibromyalgia. These events may also damage certain amino acids. In fact, emotional and physical trauma are thought to play a leading role in not only altering amino acids but also in increasing the levels of the stress hormones.

Other possible causes

Overly high stress hormone levels are capable of irritating and inflaming the intestinal lining, causing it to not function properly. The intestinal lining is intended only to allow the absorption of nutrients into the bloodstream, while keeping back toxins. Where stress hormones have indirectly caused damage to the intestinal lining, toxins are able to leak into the bloodstream. Cortisol, for example, one of the main stress hormones, interferes with sleep, which, in turn, has the effect of reducing the body's ability to repair the gut. This situation is commonly known as 'leaky gut'. The immune system then sends out antibodies to gobble up toxins it does not recognize, which may simply be large particles of food. In fibromyalgia, the immune system appears to be permanently on overdrive to deal with the leaked toxins – a weakened immune system being the eventual result.

Where fibromyalgia develops gradually over many years, as occurs in some cases, genetic factors are believed to be responsible – that is, in addition to borderline function of the amino acid transport proteins. When amino acid transport is further damaged by junk food diets, environmental chemicals, chronic exposure to the low-level toxicity found in food additives, as well as mercury vapour from amalgam tooth fillings, fibromyalgia can arise.

However, fibromyalgia symptoms are known to recede when the gut is cleaned up. The 'cleansing' process chiefly consists of:

- a detoxification programme;
- an additive-free diet;
- antioxidant-containing foods and supplementation.

This book outlines all of the above.

5

Essential nutrients

There are many nutrients essential to good health, ones that support the repair and regeneration of the tissues and cells. They fall into several categories, including vitamins, minerals, essential fatty acids, amino acids and enzymes. Enzymes are made up of vitamins and minerals and act as powerful antioxidants.

Antioxidants

Unfortunately, oxygen is not always a beneficial agent. A car needs a mixture of oxygen and fuel to run, but it is oxygen that plays a crucial role in the rusting process, shortening the life of the vehicle. Oxygen is essential to many functions within living organisms, too, and, like rust to the car, the presence of electrically unstable oxygen atoms within our bodies can seriously affect our health and longevity.

These unstable oxygen atoms – known as 'free radicals' – run riot around our bodies, damaging cell walls and important DNA. Researchers have found that disease is directly influenced by the number of free radicals present in an individual. In some instances, free radicals will cause disease, in others they will exacerbate a pre-existing illness. Antioxidants are important because they mop up free radicals.

As people with fibromyalgia are burdened with a large supply of destructive free radicals – a situation known as 'oxidative stress' – it is vital that plenty of antioxidant-containing foods, supplemented with antioxidant nutrients, are consumed. Many vitamins and minerals contain antioxidant properties, each type having its own working domain and mode of operation. The best vitamin sources include selenium, vitamin A, vitamin C and vitamin E. Good antioxidant foods are garlic, curcumine, turmeric and grapeseed extract products (proanthocyanidins – further sources are given later in this chapter).

Smoking cigarettes or cigars greatly increases free radical damage because smokers have low levels of antioxidant nutrients in their bodies. Although the above antioxidants, when taken daily, can reduce the damage caused by free radicals, the best option is to give up smoking.

Another happy outcome of consuming the recommended daily amount of antioxidants is a longer life. When bombarded with free radicals, our cells become depleted of energy – a situation that commonly leads to chronic disease, such as fibromyalgia. Eventually, the attacked cells die, which is detrimental to the individual. However, antioxidants enable our cells to be more productive, effectively preventing cell death.

In order to secure optimum functioning of each of the millions of cells in our bodies, it is important to protect them by means of a steady intake of antioxidant foods and nutritional supplements (see below for further information).

Vitamins

Unlike proteins, carbohydrates and fats, vitamins do not provide energy, nor act as building materials. Their chief function is to sustain and regulate certain biochemical processes, including cellular reproduction, digestion and the metabolic rate.

Vitamins are organic food substances found only in plants and animals. They are essential to the normal functioning of our bodies, so we must ensure that our intake of them is adequate. However, due to the use of chemicals in the production of crops, it is difficult to acquire sufficient amounts, even from a good-quality, balanced diet. The common habit of overcooking vegetables leads to a further loss in their nutritional value. In addition, people with fibromyalgia are known to suffer multiple vitamin deficiencies. It is important, therefore, that vitamin supplements are taken daily. These generally come in tablet or capsule form and can be purchased at healthfood shops and specialist suppliers. They should be taken before meals to ensure maximum absorption.

I have included the recommended daily allowance (RDA) of both vitamins and minerals for people with fibromyalgia. Although they are rather higher than the government RDAs, the latter are meant only to prevent deficiency symptoms in healthy people. However, if you suffer adverse effects from taking the amounts recommended here for fibromyalgia, reduce the dose accordingly.

Vitamin C

One of the more potent antioxidants, vitamin C aids in maintaining healthy bones, teeth and gums; wound-healing; the absorption of iron in the gut; stress hormone production and immune system function.

Vitamin C is used up in the body by smoking, alcohol consumption, surgery, trauma, stress, exposure to pollutants and the use of certain medications.

Fibromyalgia-friendly food sources are citrus fruits, strawberries, blackcurrants, tomatoes, broccoli, Brussels sprouts, cabbage, green melons, potatoes and peppers (capsicums).

As this vitamin is easily destroyed by heat and a lot of processing, it is recommended that vegetables be steamed or microwaved for as short a period of time as possible.

Vitamin C deficiency is characterized by various symptoms, including bleeding gums, swollen and/or painful joints, nosebleeds, loss of appetite, muscular weakness, slow-healing wounds, anaemia and impaired digestion.

The government recommended daily amount (RDA) is 60 mg. However, the RDA for people with fibromyalgia is 1000–2000 mg.

Vitamin A (beta-carotene – the precursor to retinol)

Also a powerful antioxidant, vitamin A is necessary for the growth and repair of the body's tissues. In addition, it reduces susceptibility to infections in the nose, mouth, throat and lungs; aids bone and teeth formation and helps to protect against pollutants.

Fibromyalgia-friendly food sources are yellow and orange fruits and vegetables, such as carrots, sweet potatoes, apricots, cantaloupe, papaya, pumpkin, melon and mango. Beta-carotene can also be found in dark, leafy vegetables, such as spinach, broccoli, cabbage and parsley.

Symptoms of deficiency are a susceptibility to infections; rough, dry, scaly skin; loss of smell and appetite; fatigue; defective teeth and gums and retarded growth.

Vitamin A should not be taken during pregnancy.

The RDA is 3333 IUs (international units) for males and 2667 IUs for females. However, the RDA for fibromyalgia is 10,000 IUs.

Vitamin E

Another major antioxidant, vitamin E assists the supply of oxygen to all the organs in the body, helping to alleviate fatigue. It also nourishes the cells, strengthens capillary walls, protects red blood cells from toxins and aids in the maintenance of nerve and muscle function.

As with other supplements, people taking warfarin should check with their doctor before taking vitamin E supplements.

Fibromyalgia-friendly food sources are mostly oil, seed and grain derivatives. These include wheatgerm, safflower, avocados, sunflower oil and seeds, pumpkin seeds, linseeds, almonds, Brazil nuts, cashews, pecans, wholegrain cereals and breads, wheatgerm, asparagus, dried prunes and broccoli.

Symptoms of vitamin E deficiency are dry skin; red blood cell rupture; decline in sexual vitality; abnormal fat deposits in the muscles; degenerative changes in the heart and the muscles and the onset of autoimmune disease (fibromyalgia is an autoimmune disease – 'autoimmune' means that the immune system is confused into attacking healthy tissues, such as the muscles, ligaments and tendons).

The RDA is 10 mg, but, for those with fibromyalgia, it is 250 mg.

B complex vitamins

As the B vitamins are required at every stage of energy manufacture, and because they assist in the calming process and in maintaining good mental health, a regular intake is required in the treatment of fibromyalgia. B vitamins are also integral to the production of serotonin, the pain-reducing, sleep-promoting hormone that fibromyalgics have in short supply. For all these reasons, B complex vitamin supplements are highly recommended for people with fibromyalgia. Avoid taking them at night, however, as they may interfere with sleep.

Vitamin B1 (thiamine)

This vitamin is essential for blood cell metabolism; muscle metabolism; digestion; pain inhibition and energy production, all of which can be problem areas in fibromyalgia. In fact, people with fibromyalgia are known to exhibit a low vitamin B1 status, causing reduced activity of the thiamine-dependent enzymes. A diet that is low in sugars and high in wholegrains will improve vitamin B levels, however.

Fibromyalgia-friendly food sources are oatmeal, whole wheat, brown rice, bran, wheatgerm, lentils, lean meats, free-range eggs, dried beans, sunflower seeds and peanuts. Herbs containing B1 are peppermint, slippery elm, ginseng, gotu kola and kelp.

Deficiency problems include burning and tingling in the toes and soles of the feet, depression, fatigue, muscle weakness, difficulty sleeping, irritability and loss of appetite.

The RDA is 1.5 mg for males and 1.1 mg for females. However, the RDA for fibromyalgia is 30 mg.

Vitamin B2 (riboflavin)

Necessary for red blood formation; cell respiration; antibody formation and fat and carbohydrate metabolism, the body should be supplied with vitamin B2 daily. Levels of this vitamin in the body can be reduced by caffeine, alcohol and some antibiotics.

Fibromyalgia-friendly food sources are peanuts, free-range eggs, lean meats, soya products, whole grains and leafy green vegetables.

Deficiency symptoms include insomnia; dry, cracked lips; a red, scaly nose; gritty eyes, sore lips and tongue and photophobia (light-sensitive eyes).

The RDA is 1.7 mg for males and 1.3 mg for females. However, the RDA for fibromyalgia is 25 mg.

Vitamin B3 (niacinamide)

This vitamin is necessary for the production of several hormones, including insulin, female and male hormones and thyroxine, the hormone produced by the thyroid gland. It is also involved in blood circulation, acid production, histamine activation and conversion of carbohydrates to energy.

Fibromyalgia-friendly food sources are white meat, whole wheat, oily fish, avocados, nuts, peanuts, sunflower seeds, whole grains and prunes.

B3 deficiency can cause hypoglycaemia, confusion, memory loss, irritability, diarrhoea, depression, fatigue, muscle weakness, insomnia and ringing in the ears.

The RDA is 1.1 mg. However, the RDA for fibromyalgia is 100 mg.

Vitamin B5 (pantothenic acid)

The adrenal glands, which sit on top of the kidneys, can be damaged by stress, causing 'adrenal exhaustion' and all manner of problems. Further damage can be prevented, however, by taking this supplement. B5 is also crucial to the release of energy from protein, carbohydrates, fats and sugars; for the production of the anti-stress hormones and for good health of the nervous system.

Symptoms of deficiency include muscle pain; dizzy spells; skin abnormalities; digestive problems; poor muscle coordination, restlessness; fatigue, depression and insomnia.

Fibromyalgia-friendly food sources are whole grains, soft-boiled egg yolk, fish, brewer's yeast, peanuts, walnuts, dried pears and apricots, dates and mushrooms.

The RDA is 6 mg. However, the RDA for fibromyalgia is 50 mg.

Vitamin B6 (pyridoxine)

Needed for the conversion of fats and proteins into energy, vitamin B6 is vital for correct balance in the body and important for those who suffer excessive stress. It also aids in the production of serotonin, and is essential for magnesium metabolism – both of which fibromyalgics have in short supply.

Symptoms of B6 deficiency include nervousness, depression, muscle weakness, pain, headaches, irritability, stiff joints and PMS in women.

Fibromyalgia-friendly food sources are bananas, wholegrain bread, lean meats, eggs, dried beans, avocados, seeds, nuts, chicken, fish and liver.

The RDA is 2 mg. Although the safety of vitamin B6 supplementation has been under the spotlight in recent years, the fibromyalgia RDA of 50 mg is considered safe, even for long-term use.

Vitamin B12 (cobalamin)

This vitamin is crucial to protein, carbohydrate and fat metabolism, red blood cell formation and longevity of cells. As B12 is found in animal products, supplementation is essential for vegans. Muscle weakness, fatigue, depression, paranoia, memory loss and headaches are symptoms of vitamin B12 deficiency.

Fibromyalgia-friendly food sources are soft-boiled egg yolk, fish, shellfish, lean meats and poultry.

The RDA is 1 mcg. However, the RDA for fibromyalgia is 250 mcg.

Vitamin D

Known as the 'forgotten vitamin', vitamin D aids calcium absorption and helps to form and maintain strong bones. It also works in concert with a number of other vitamins, minerals and hormones to promote bone mineralization. Without vitamin D, the bones can become thin, brittle or misshapen (see page 14 for information about osteoporosis). Research also indicates that vitamin D helps to maintain a healthy immune system and assists in regulating cell growth and differentiation – the process that determines what a cell is to become.

A deficiency of vitamin D is now believed to be a major cause of unexplained muscle and bone pain. Indeed, in a study of 150 children and adults with unexplained musculo-skeletal pain, almost all were found to be severely deficient in this vitamin. A later study found that volunteers with pain were also vitamin D deficient, regardless of their ages. Research released by the American Society of Anesthesiologists has shown that a quarter of people with chronic pain have low levels of vitamin D in the blood. Researchers from the Mayo Comprehensive Pain Rehabilitation Center found that, out of 267 adults undergoing morphine treatment for chronic pain. 26 per cent had a vitamin D deficiency, which was also associated with lower levels of physical functioning, poor overall health and an increased requirement for morphine. Cancers of the prostate, colon and breast are also linked with vitamin D deficiency, as are heart disease and auto-immune diseases such as rheumatoid arthritis and even type 1 diabetes.

One 2014 study, led by Dr Florian Wepner of the Orthopaedic Hospital, Vienna, Austria, found that vitamin D supplements helped relieve pain and morning fatigue in people with fibromyalgia, especially those with low levels of calcifediol, a pre-hormone produced in the liver which is then converted to the active form of vitamin D. A 2012 Saudi Arabian study of 30 women with fibromyalgia, published in the journal *Pain Medicine*, found that people with fibromyalgia tended to be deficient in vitamin D. The results also indicated that treatment with high-dose vitamin D3 resulted in significant improvement of most fibromyalgia symptoms.

It is possible to obtain vitamin D from foods and supplements, but this is not easy. A glass of fortified milk or orange juice contains about 100 IUs of vitamin D, whereas a multivitamin typically holds about 400 IUs. However, the RDA for fibromyalgia and unexplained pain is between 200 and 1000 IUs, depending on your age, sex and medical condition. Other sources of vitamin D are cod liver oil (1 tbsp equals 1360 IU of vitamin D); salmon (75 g (3 oz) equals 425 IU of vitamin D); herring 75 g (3 oz) equals 765 IU of vitamin D, and canned sardines 75 g (3 oz) equals 255 IU of vitamin D.

However, we tend to obtain most of our vitamin D from exposure to sunlight. Therefore, people who seldom venture outdoors or always wear sunscreen are at risk of vitamin D deficiency. The message that all unprotected sun exposure is bad for you is too extreme. Indeed, experts now believe that a few minutes daily of unprotected sun exposure is important for health.

Low vitamin D levels are not in themselves thought to cause fibromyalgia, but they are associated with continued or increased disease activity. Previous studies have found that vitamin D deficiency is associated with anxiety and depression in fibromyalgia. Indeed, some doctors believe that vitamin D deficiency is misdiagnosed as fibromyalgia (see Table 3.1).

Table 3.1 Spot the difference – vitamin D deficiency and fibromyalgia symptoms

Can your doctor tell the difference? If not, don't blame him or her – the symptoms are very similar.

Vitamin D deficiency symptoms	Fibromyalgia symptoms
Muscle pain	Widespread pain
Weakness	Muscle tenderness
Bone pain	Fatigue
Fractures	Depression and anxiety
Fatigue/lack of energy	Difficulty sleeping
Low mood, depression	Irritable bowel syndrome (IBS)
Mood swings	
Difficulty sleeping	
Digestive problems	

Vitamin P (bioflavonoids and proanthocyanidins)

Because they work with vitamin C, bioflavonoids are essential for people with fibromyalgia. The condition means that the cells allow substances to leak through thin blood vessel walls to accumulate in tissues where they are not supposed to be. Natural plant bioflavonoids, such as rutin, hesperidin and quercetin, help to strengthen the vessels and capillaries. High-potency bioflavonoids called 'proanthocyanidins' – the most potent of which is grape-seed extract (available from healthfood shops and specialist suppliers) – also strengthen the blood vessels and capillaries. Their other benefits include strengthening connective tissues and muscle fibre; enhancing muscle fibre function; improving the energy production process and reducing free radical damage. They also assist in utilizing other nutrients.

Although they are found in virtually all plant foods, the best fibromyalgia-friendly food sources are fresh fruit and vegetables, legumes, whole grains, seeds, nuts, spinach, apricots, cherries, rosehips, grapes, blackberries and tea. Bioflavonoid-containing herbs include paprika and rosehips. Milk thistle seed, ginkgo biloba and pycnogenol (which is obtained from grapeseed extract) are high in bioflavonoids and can be purchased in tablet form from healthfood shops and specialist suppliers.

There is no government RDA for bioflavonoids and proanthocyanidins as they are groups of nutrients. People with fibromyalgia should try to consume the above foods and take milk thistle and ginkgo biloba supplements, closely following the dosage instructions on the container (more about milk thistle and ginkgo biloba under 'Other useful supplements' later in this chapter).

Biotin

This vitamin reduces stress, aids nutrient absorption and is especially beneficial to individuals who eat a poor-quality diet. It helps protein, carbohydrate and fat metabolism; cell growth; fatty acid production and energy metabolism.

Biotin deficiency is characterized by muscle pain, fatigue, depression, nausea, anaemia, hair loss, anorexia, dermatitis and high cholesterol levels.

Fibromyalgia-friendly food sources are lean meats, soft-boiled egg yolk and whole grains.

The RDA is 150 mcg. However, the RDA for fibromyalgia is 400 mcg.

Minerals

Minerals are our most essential nutrients. The body requires small amounts of a wide range of minerals on a daily basis to ensure the normal functioning of all its systems. Carbohydrates, fats, vitamins, enzymes and amino acids all require minerals for their particular operations. However, one of their more important functions is that of aiding the regulation of the delicate balance of bodily fluids. They are also essential to the process of waste elimination and for bringing oxygen and nutrients to the cells.

As minerals continue to disappear from our soils, human beings face an ongoing rise in mineral deficiencies. In addition, government studies have shown that prolonged stress and anxiety can lead to mineral imbalances, which is now considered a major factor in the onset of fibromyalgia.

People with fibromyalgia are known to have abnormally low levels of magnesium and manganese. Many sufferers also have other mineral deficiencies and, unfortunately, a shortfall of essential minerals causes deficiencies in protein and vitamins. Besides eating a quality, well-balanced diet, it is imperative that people with fibromyalgia take mineral supplements. These usually come in tablet form and can be purchased at healthfood shops, pharmacies and the larger supermarkets.

It is important to be aware that all minerals are bound to something else, which is known as 'chelation', and the amount of mineral absorbed by the body depends on what the mineral is chelated to.

'Inorganic chelates' are naturally occurring mined minerals that are not easily absorbed. For example, women with osteoporosis may take calcium carbonate. However, its absorption may be as little as 5 per cent – that's 50 mg from a 1000 mg supplement. Oxides, sulphates and phosphates are also inorganic chelates and may not be very useful.

'Organic chelates', on the other hand, can achieve up to 60 per cent absorption. So, while the milligrams figure may be lower, the body will absorb far greater amounts. Check the label for the words 'amino acid chelate', 'citrate', 'picolinate' or 'glycinate', which indicate that the product is an organic chelate. Also, see Vitamin D, above, for details of how to obtain this important aid to calcium absorption. Because organic chelated minerals are more expensive to produce, the cost to the consumer is greater than that of their inorganic counterparts. However, the cost is more than made up for by their far superior effects.

The following are important minerals:

Calcium

This vital mineral is the most abundant in the body – 99 per cent of it being found in the bones and teeth. Calcium works to tighten and constrict bodily tissues, including the bones, whereas its sister, magnesium, exerts a relaxing effect. In fact, calcium and magnesium work together to ensure proper muscle contraction and relaxation as well as the building of muscle fibres and connective tissues. Calcium also builds and maintains strong bones and teeth, is involved in the regulation of heart rhythm, aids the passage of nutrients into cell walls, assists in normal blood clotting, helps maintain normal blood pressure and is essential to normal kidney function.

A deficiency in calcium is common and can be signalled by muscle cramps; tingling in the lips, fingers and feet; leg numbness; tooth decay; sensitivity to noise; depression and deterioration of the bones (osteoporosis). Too much calcium, however, is known to be implicated in bone brittleness, whereas sufficient magnesium intake will allow the bones the necessary 'give' to counteract jarring and sudden impacts.

Fibromyalgia-friendly food sources are dried peas, tinned sardines and salmon (including the bones), oranges, nuts, seeds, root vegetables and leafy green vegetables. As a low dairy diet is advisable for people with fibromyalgia, a magnesium/calcium/zinc supplement should make up the shortfall.

The RDA is 800 mg. However, the RDA for fibromyalgia is 1000 mg.

Magnesium

This important mineral aids the absorption of calcium, phosphorus, potassium, vitamins C and E, and the B complex vitamins. It is integral to the regulation and maintenance of normal heart activity; it helps to make bones less prone to breakage, and, together with calcium and vitamin C, aids the conversion of blood sugar into energy.

Magnesium deficiency is as common as that of calcium and, due to the precarious balance between these two associated minerals, deficiency can also be caused by excessive calcium supplementation. Junk foods are frequently low in magnesium, and processed bran added to a poor diet can render magnesium useless. Deficiency symptoms include muscle pain and tenderness; fatigue; migraine and headaches; tremor and shakiness; poor mental function, allergies, palpitations and numbness and tingling in the fingers and toes.

As it appears that all fibromyalgics suffer magnesium deficiencies, supplementation is highly recommended.

Fibromyalgia-friendly food sources include whole grains, leafy green vegetables, nuts – especially almonds and cashews – seeds, legumes, tofu and soya products, vegetables – especially broccoli and sweetcorn, bananas and apricots.

The RDA is 270 mg. However, the RDA for fibromyalgia is 600 mg. (See 'The importance of a magnesium and malic acid combination' on pages 46–7.)

Manganese

Part of an important antioxidant enzyme system, manganese plays a vital role in fibromyalgia. It helps create energy from glucose and aids in the normalization of the central nervous system. It is also essential for normal skeletal development; activates enzymes known to be helpful in the digestion and utilization of foods, and plays a key role in the breakdown of fats and cholesterol.

Deficiency symptoms include digestive problems, dizziness, paralysis and convulsions.

Fibromyalgia-friendly food sources are leafy green vegetables, whole grains, nuts, seeds and tea.

The RDA for fibromyalgia is 10 mg.

Zinc

Another important antioxidant, zinc is involved in blood stability; wound-healing; protein synthesis, digestion and the development and maintenance of the reproductive organs. This mineral is often low in Western diets. Vegetarian diets may be especially deficient – the high grain content binds the zinc, rendering it useless. This mineral is also crucial to growth and development; hair and nail growth; the formation of skin and insulin output.

Zinc should be accompanied by copper in a ratio of 10–15 mg of zinc to 1 mg of copper, to prevent a possible copper imbalance.

Deficiency symptoms include white spots on the finger nails, stretch marks, fatigue, decreased alertness, susceptibility to infections and delayed sexual maturity.

Fibromyalgia-friendly food sources are the herbs liquorice and ginseng, oysters, lean meats, liver, wheatgerm, pumpkin seeds and sunflower seeds.

The RDA is 15 mg and people with fibromyalgia require approximately this amount.

Selenium

A major antioxidant, this mineral protects cells from the toxic effects of free radicals and, in so doing, boosts the immune system. In the process of oxidation, selenium slows down the ageing and hardening of tissues and preserves tissue elasticity. It is also beneficial for the prevention and treatment of dandruff.

Selenium deficiency symptoms include premature ageing, loose skin, dandruff and heart disease.

Fibromyalgia-friendly food sources are tuna, salmon, shrimps, garlic, tomatoes, sunflower seeds, Brazil nuts and wheat breads.

The RDA for fibromyalgia is 100 mcg.

Potassium

This mineral works with sodium to regulate heart and muscle function. It also ensures the normal transmission of nerve impulses; aids normal growth; stimulates the kidneys to eliminate toxic body waste; and promotes healthy skin.

Deficiency symptoms include poor reflexes, muscle twitches, weakness and soreness, nervous disorders, erratic and/or rapid heartbeats, insomnia, fatigue and high cholesterol levels.

Fibromyalgia-friendly food sources are bananas, lean meats, avocados, tomato juice, fruit juice, nuts, salad vegetables, potatoes, oranges and dried fruits.

The RDA is 3500 mg. However, the RDA for fibromyalgia is 5000 mg.

Chromium

Chromium is part of what is known as the 'glucose tolerance factor', which means that it helps the body to metabolize sugar and stabilize blood sugar levels. It also increases the efficiency of insulin in metabolizing carbohydrates.

Chromium deficiency is indicated by weight loss, glucose intolerance, tiredness, diabetes and heart disease.

Fibromyalgia-friendly food sources are brewer's yeast, mushrooms, wheatgerm and low-fat cheese.

The RDA for fibromyalgia is 200 mcg.

Other useful supplements

Malic acid

As it is essential for energy production, malic acid is of prime importance in the treatment of fibromyalgia. It is also vital for reducing the toxic effects of aluminium – a scourge in autoimmune diseases such as fibromyalgia.

When combined with magnesium, malic acid can be particularly effective, so some supplement manufacturers now offer 'magnesium malate', which combines the two. (See 'The importance of a magnesium and malic acid combination' on pages 46–7.)

Fibromyalgia-friendly food sources are all fruits, but apples have by far the highest content.

The RDA for fibromyalgia is 200 mg.

5-Hydroxytryptophan (5-HTP)

Because of its ability to increase serotonin levels, this phytonutrient (plant derivative) is known to be useful for treating fibromyalgia. Its benefits include pain, anxiety and fatigue reduction. It is also known to improve sleep.

The RDA for fibromyalgics is 100–500 mg daily, depending on the individual (see also Chapter 4). As with all other supplements, please consult your doctor before starting 5-HTP supplementation.

Glucosamine

A type of nutrient known as an 'amino sugar', glucosamine governs the number of water-holding molecules in cartilage and is converted to larger molecules that make up connective tissue. This nutrient is now known to be effective in reducing the effects of arthritic conditions. In a study known as the Vulvodynia Project, led by Dr C. C. Solomons in Denver, Colorado, in 1997, it successfully decreased pain and sensitivity in the soft tissues (muscles, ligaments and tendons) of subjects with fibromyalgia.

Available only as a nutritional supplement, it is often combined with vitamin C and the amino acid tyrosine to maximize its action. The RDA for fibromyalgia is 1000 mg.

Boron

This trace element is important in maintaining good muscular health. It is also believed to reduce calcium loss in postmenopausal women.

Deficiency symptoms are thought to include osteoporosis and menopausal symptoms in women.

Fibromyalgia-friendly food sources are apples, pears, prunes, seeds, raisins, tomatoes and cauliflower.

The RDA for fibromyalgia is 3 mg.

Co-enzyme Q10

This enzyme aids the transfer of oxygen and energy between components of the cells and between the blood and the tissues. It is highly beneficial to people with nutritional deficiencies, such as fibromyalgia sufferers.

Fibromyalgia-friendly food sources are peanuts and other nuts, mackerel, chicken, whole grains, sardines and spinach.

Co-enzyme Q10 (also known as coQ10) can be purchased in capsule form from healthfood shops and specialist supplement suppliers.

The RDA for fibromyalgia is 100 mg. Your doctor should be consulted before you begin co-enzyme Q10 supplementation.

DHEA (dehydroepiandosterone)

Secreted by the adrenal glands, DHEA is one of the most abundant hormones in the body. Its use has shown great benefits for immune system disorders, such as fibromyalgia, osteoporosis and chronic fatigue syndrome. However, DHEA is produced naturally when good nutrition occurs. This hormone may only be obtained on prescription from your doctor.

Ginkgo biloba

The effectiveness of ginkgo biloba is now well documented. When used in the treatment of fibromyalgia, this herbal antioxidant can help maintain and support the body's circulation, particularly to the extremities – the hands and feet and, most importantly, the brain. The advantages include better cerebral blood flow; improved tissue oxygenation; more efficient energy production; and improved cognitive function – that is, concentration and short-term memory.

In two trials undertaken in the 1990s, volunteers were given ginkgo biloba daily. The first trial[3] showed that their short-term memories had improved significantly and, in the second,[4] the volunteers displayed even sharper reactions and better memories, as well as improved brain function – all of which were judged to be due to improved circulation. Ginkgo biloba is, therefore, considered very useful in the treatment of fibromyalgia.

This herb can be purchased in capsule form from healthfood shops, chemists and the larger supermarkets. The dosage instructions given on the label should be closely followed. As people on prescription medication – warfarin and aspirin, for example – can react adversely to ginkgo biloba, please consult your doctor before taking this supplement.

Milk thistle

Milk thistle not only protects the liver from disease and damage due to ingested or inhaled toxins, it is also capable of regenerating damaged liver tissue. Unfortunately, though, it is ineffective when brewed into a tea.

Milk thistle can be purchased in capsule form and the label dosage instructions should be followed. Again, please consult your doctor before taking this herbal supplement.

Oil of evening primrose

This essential fatty acid of the omega 6 family is extracted from the seed of the evening primrose plant. It contains a percentage of gamma linolenic acid or GLA – a vital link in prostaglandin manufacture. (Prostaglandins are hormone-like substances involved in reducing inflammation in the body. They are also involved in blood clotting, blood pressure and hormone regulation.) However, conversion of linolenic acid (omega 6) to GLA can be slowed down by foods rich in saturated fat, alcohol, excessive sugar, zinc deficiency, stress and ageing. When omega 6 conversion to GLA is inefficient, supplementation is highly recommended.

Oil of evening primrose is often taken by women prior to menstruation to help maintain GLA levels. Because it aids hormone balance, it is also recommended for people with fibromyalgia.

The RDA is 500–1000 mg.

Some important points to remember about RDAs

In most instances, the recommended daily amounts (RDAs) of vitamin and mineral supplements set by the Department of Health are only intended to prevent common diseases associated with a severe deficiency. They are not intended to promote the optimal functioning and protection of bodily systems. RDAs, therefore, are the very minimum intake required for good health. For example, the RDA for vitamin E is 10 mg, but scientific research has shown that the level offering protection to the heart is in excess of 67 mg. Of course, this amount is inclusive of vitamin E obtained from natural sources.

The importance of a magnesium and malic acid combination

Supplements of magnesium and malic acid – also formulated as magnesium malate – are believed to markedly reduce the pain and fatigue of fibromyalgia.

As stated earlier, magnesium is essential to many bodily functions. However, it plays a vital role in the operation of the important malic acid shuttle service, which delivers vital nutrients to the cells. Malic acid enters the cycle at the most efficient site and is then converted into usable energy. As a component of what is known as the Kreb's cycle, malic acid also deals with the build-up of lactic acid in the muscles and other soft tissues.

In a study carried out in 1992,[5] fibromyalgia volunteers were given 6 to 12 tablets a day containing a magnesium and malic acid combination, each tablet consisting of 50 mg of magnesium and 200 mg of malic acid. After four weeks, their pain levels were halved. After a further four weeks, they fell even more – from an initial pain score of 19.6, down to 6.5. For the next two weeks, six patients were then switched to a placebo (a sugar pill with no active ingredients, but the patients are not told this so they think they are taking medicine). Their pain scores rose from 6.5 to 21.5, the pain and fatigue distinctly worsening within 48 hours of switching to the placebo.

In a later study,[6] fibromyalgia volunteers were not informed whether they were taking the supplements or a placebo. The findings of the first study were confirmed, with the clarification that only patients taking at least six magnesium and malic acid combination supplements a day showed a significant reduction in pain.

Magnesium and malic acid appear to reduce the pain issuing from the 'trigger points' found in fibromyalgia – these being specific sites from which pain radiates to other parts of the body.

To achieve the desired effect, you should take six 75-mg magnesium tablets a day (450 mg) for eight to ten months to raise your levels to normal, then two tablets a day (150 mg) to maintain the improvement. A dose of 300 mg of malic acid – that is, 100 mg, taken three times a day – should be followed initially, dropping to a maintenance level of 100 mg daily after eight to ten months.

Magnesium and malic acid supplements may be bought separately or else combined in the form of magnesium malate (see the Useful addresses section at the back of the book for recommended supplement manufacturers and distributors). However, you would be advised to consult your doctor before embarking on this treatment. Diarrhoea is a possible side-effect.

Guidance on taking supplements

Studies have shown that vitamins A, C and E (known as the 'ACE' vitamins), together with co-enzyme Q10, selenium, zinc and manganese supplements, work as fine antioxidants, reducing the oxidative stress of fibromyalgia and aiding the healing process. These substances may be purchased together in a single antioxidant supplement from certain health supplement manufacturers, and are sold under different brand names (see the Useful addresses section at the back of the book for details of recommended supplement manufacturers). Alternatively the constituents may be bought separately, but generally at a higher price. Trials have shown that the above-mentioned combination of supplements should be taken for a period of one month before commencing further radical supplementation. However, evening primrose oil and B complex supplementation could be started after two weeks. Remember that it is important to take sufficient vitamin B5 (pantothenic acid).

During month two, I would suggest that you begin magnesium and malic acid supplementation. As you will recall, these work together to reduce pain, fatigue and low muscle stamina, but, in the main, can only be bought separately (see the Useful addresses section, however, for details of manufacturers who produce a combination supplement). A multimineral supplement containing calcium, manganese, zinc, boron and magnesium should also be taken.

During months three and four, it would be helpful to begin taking 5-HTP, together with ginkgo biloba, co-enzyme Q10, glucosamine and milk thistle. All of these work in different ways to improve the symptoms of fibromyalgia.

I appreciate that a fair amount of expenditure is called for to do this, but, because of the many deficiencies in fibromyalgia, supplementation is very important. Apart from following a healthy diet, there is, to date, no better way to significantly reduce your symptoms. By following the diet alone, you should make a noticeable difference to your health, but, by incorporating the recommended supplements into your regime, you will give your body an even greater chance of healing. Having said that, please remember that to take only one or two types of supplements is better than taking none at all. The antioxidant supplements are of prime importance, as is the magnesium and malic acid (magnesium malate) supplement.

As we are all very different, I would advise that you test the effects of each supplement to assess the required dosage for you, maybe even commencing each type of supplement separately to more accurately judge its effects. You may actually require a higher or lower dosage than initially supposed. High levels should, however, be reduced to maintenance levels after eight to ten months.

Because there is some doubt as to the amounts of certain supplements needed to treat fibromyalgia, you may prefer to consult a nutritionist. He or she will not only advise you about correct dosages but also give clear and careful guidance regarding your diet.

6

Substances to avoid

Although I have already outlined the dangers of chemically grown produce and toxic food additives, there are, unfortunately, many more inhospitable foods and substances that ultimately suppress our immune systems and cause other damage. People with fibromyalgia are particularly susceptible to the effects of such substances.

Stimulants

Our bodies need rest and relaxation in order to function at optimum levels. When these are withheld, high stress levels make us crave stimulants to help us continue to function. Alcohol, cigarettes, caffeine-containing products, such as coffee, tea, cocoa and chocolate, and products containing refined white sugar, such as cakes, biscuits and sweets, provide an energy 'lift'. They stimulate our systems. Unfortunately, not only is the lift short-lived, leaving us feeling lower than before in its wake, these substances are also known to be detrimental to our health.

The elimination of stimulants should bring about improvements in every area in fibromyalgia – particularly where energy levels and anxiety are concerned. If you find that you are unable to completely eliminate stimulants from your diet, however, reduce them as much as possible – it will make a difference.

In general, you may find this diet easier to adhere to if you allow yourself an occasional treat. Try to beware letting the treats become routine, however! Obviously the strategy for smoking is different. If you manage to cut out smoking, an occasional cigarette will risk undoing all your hard work.

Caffeine

Caffeine products can not only cause stress to the adrenal glands, they are also toxic to the liver. In addition they can reduce the body's ability to absorb vitamins and minerals. Caffeine is addictive, too – it has cocaine, morphine, strychnine, nicotine and atropine as close family members and all of these are nerve poisons. Consumed regularly, coffee and other caffeine-containing products, such as tea, chocolate, cocoa and cola drinks, are also likely to give rise to chronic anxiety – the symptoms of which are agitation, palpitations, headaches, indigestion, panic, insomnia and hyper-ventilation. Chronic anxiety is a symptom commonly occurring with fibromyalgia. However, it is the toxicity of caffeine that may contribute to the development of fibromyalgia. My best advice is to remove caffeine products from your diet.

Unfortunately, because caffeine is addictive, reducing intake is far from easy. Withdrawal symptoms can take the form of splitting headaches, fatigue, depression, poor concentration and muscle pains. It is no wonder people can feel terrible until they have had their first dose of caffeine in the morning and that they cannot seem to function properly without regular doses throughout the day!

Caffeine is 'washed out' of the system very quickly, however, so it is possible to minimize withdrawal symptoms by gradually reducing your intake over several weeks. Believe me, when it has been totally removed from your system, you certainly feel the difference!

Sugar

It has been said that after stress, alcohol and drugs, sugar poses the greatest risk to health in the Western world. It is added to almost all processed and pre-prepared foods and has a drug-like effect on the body. A couple of biscuits or a slice of cake will provide us with an instant lift, but to the detriment of our long-term health. Sugar fills us up in place of the foods our bodies need. Furthermore, it has no nutritional value, providing us with empty calories that only cause us to put on weight via insulin, the fat-storage hormone.

Many years ago, Stone Age people only had access to the unrefined sugars present in fruit – 'unrefined' meaning not having undergone any form of processing. The only refined sugar available to them was honey, but their digestive systems were able to handle this occasional excess. Nowadays, many refined sugars are available to us, but, unfortunately, our bodies have not progressed enough to enable us to cope with them efficiently.

It does not help that modern people have trained themselves to have a sweet tooth. There are alternatives to sugar, however. For example, you can sweeten your drinks and desserts by adding fresh fruit, or baked apples by sprinkling on cinnamon.

Here are some alternatives to refined white sugar. By 'a cup' is meant a teacup or American measure, not a mug.

- **Honey** Raw, unprocessed honey is high in enzymes. Half a cup of honey replaces one cup of refined white sugar.
- **Fructose** The sugar from fruit – fructose – resembles white table sugar but, like sugar, it is of no nutritional value. As it requires processing by the liver, it should be used in moderation. Half a cup of fructose replaces one cup of refined white sugar.
- **Muscovado** Muscovado sugar is the first crude crystals that appear when sugar beet and cane are processed. It is brown and sticky and contains healthy organic acids. One cup of muscovado replaces one cup of refined white sugar.
- **Molasses** The residue from the first stage of crystallization from sugar beet and cane is molasses, which is bitter and black. Like muscovado, it, too, is rich in organic acids. Half a cup of molasses replaces one cup of refined white sugar.
- **Demerara sugar or soft brown sugar or Barbados sugar** This comes from the next stage of the sugar refining process. As it has still undergone far less processing than ordinary white sugar, it contains more nutrients, including organic acids. One cup of demerara or soft brown sugar replaces one cup of refined white sugar.
- **Brown rice syrup** The slow boiling of brown rice results in a thick, honey-like syrup. One cup of brown rice syrup replaces one cup of refined white sugar.
- **Date sugar** Made from ground, dehydrated dates, date sugar has a high vitamin and mineral content. Two-thirds of a cup of date sugar replaces one cup of refined white sugar.
- **Barley malt** A syrup made from roasted barley, barley malt contains several minerals and trace amounts of the B vitamins. One cup of barley malt replaces one cup of refined white sugar.
- **Fruit juice sweetener** This is simply unprocessed fruit juice, offering all the vitamins and minerals of fruit. One cup of this sweetener replaces one cup of refined white sugar.

- **Maple syrup** Made from boiled down maple tree sap, half a cup of maple syrup replaces one cup of refined white sugar.

All the above-mentioned white sugar substitutes may be used in cooking and baking.

Alcohol

As fibromyalgia is a disorder of the central nervous system and alcohol is a nerve poison, consuming alcohol can further complicate the nerve transmission process. It may work well as an analgesic, but the effects are short-lived.

Alcohol consumption is known to deplete the B vitamins and probably antioxidants as they are required to mop up the damaging free radicals stimulated by the liver's alcohol detoxification process. In the long term, anything but very modest alcohol consumption is likely to cause more problems than it takes away. I would recommend, therefore, that it be consumed in moderation, if at all.

Even more damaging is the fact that pesticides, colourants and other harmful additives are generally involved in modern-day alcohol production, exerting further strain on the liver. If you cannot avoid the occasional drink, red wine would appear to be the best choice.

On the positive side, some researchers have found that a little tipple may do you good if you have fibromyalgia. Researchers from the Mayo Clinic in the USA and the University of Michigan found that low and moderate drinkers (3–7 drinks a week) had less fatigue and pain, and better work rates, vitality and general health, than teetotallers. Dr Terry Oh, who led this study, said,

> Aminobutyric acid (GABA), an inhibitory neurotransmitter, is low in the brain in fibromyalgia, which may go some way to explain why the nervous system reaction to pain is amplified. Alcohol binds to the GABA receptor in the central nervous system which in turn may turn down pain transmission. However the effects of alcohol may also be due to improved mood, socialization and tension, and while moderate drinkers have fewer symptoms there are still many questions about how this happens.

Tobacco

As mentioned earlier, cigarette and cigar smoking increases the number of destructive free radicals within the body. In addition, smokers have low levels of selenium and vitamins A, C and E – all of which are active antioxidants. Smokers also carry high levels of cadmium, a toxic metal, in their bodies. My best advice is to give up smoking.

Aspartame

Aspartame, a widely used artificial sweetener, is surrounded by controversy. When given to monkeys in tests it proved harmless, but that, it is now believed, is because of the highly nutritious, antioxidant-rich foods these animals consume. Experts have now drawn the conclusion that aspartame is harmless to individuals on antioxidant-rich diets, but may cause problems in people who are not.

I have now read several articles about the unwelcome side-effects of aspartame and conclude that perhaps people with fibromyalgia should 'err on the side of caution'. 'Aspartame poisoning' is said to produce many of the symptoms and conditions occurring in fibromyalgia. These include muscle spasms, shooting pains, joint pain, depression, anxiety, fatigue and weakness, headaches, sleep problems, dizziness, diarrhoea, tinnitus, mood changes, blurred vision and short-term memory loss.

People with fibromyalgia have abnormally sensitive pain receptors, thus making them more susceptible to aspartame, according to Dr Michael McNett, director of the Fibromyalgia Treatment Centers of America. A 2010 study at Dijon University Hospital found a definite link between aspartame intake and fibromyalgia, calling it 'aspartame-induced fibromyalgia, an unusual but curable cause of chronic pain'. While the study featured only two people, it found that in both cases, as soon as aspartame was given up, fibromyalgia symptoms vanished. Another small study published in the *Annals of Pharmacotherapy* found that, when patients with fibromyalgia avoided aspartame as well as monosodium glutamate (MSG), they felt better overall. It was concluded that it could be worth adding aspartame intake to the list of regular questions physicians ask their patients.

Studies have repeatedly found that artificial sweeteners such as aspartame can in fact increase weight gain as they stimulate appetite and increase carbohydrate cravings. A study published in the journal *Appetite* in 2013 cited a Brazilian study which showed that rats fed aspartame gained more weight than those fed plain sucrose – even though actual calorie intake was similar. A 2010 review published in the *Yale Journal of Biology and Medicine* looked at the neurobiology of sweet cravings and the effect of artificial sweeteners on appetite control. It examined several large studies and found a link between artificial sweeteners and weight gain. Dr H. J. Roberts, author of *Aspartame Disease: An Ignored Epidemic* (Sunshine Sentinel Press, 1999), was a pioneer in warning of the dangers of aspartame. In particular, he believed that aspartame addiction is a significant problem.

I would advise, therefore, that if the label says 'sugar free' or 'diet', check the list of additives. The brand-named aspartame products should be avoided, too.

Food additives

Up to 80 per cent of the foods on our supermarket shelves have undergone some degree of refinement or chemical alteration.

Food additives to watch out for are the following.

- **MSG** These letters stand for monosodium glutamate, which is the most common flavour enhancer on the market. As manufacturers are not required to call it MSG on the label, it is often disguised as hydrolysed yeast, autolysed yeast, yeast extract, sodium caseinate, natural flavouring, vegetable protein, hydrolysed protein, other spices, and natural chicken or turkey flavouring.
- **BHT** This is butylated hydroxyanisole, which is a widely used preservative. It is used in baked goods, breakfast cereals, potatoes, pastry mixes, dry mixes for desserts, chewing gum, sweets, ice-cream and so on. BHT can adversely affect liver and kidney function and has been associated with behavioural problems in children.
- **Sorbate** A preservative and fungus preventative, sorbate can be found in drinks, baked goods, pie fillings, artificially sweetened jellies, preserves, prepared salads and fresh fruit cocktails.
- **Sulphites** Used in bleaching and preserving certain foods, this substance prevents the discoloration of light-coloured fruit and vegetables, enabling them to look fresh for longer. Sulphites are often found in beer, lager, wine and sliced fruit. They may also be

present in packaged wine vinegar, gravies, avocado dip, sauces, potatoes and lemon juice.

- **Aspartame** Mentioned earlier in this chapter, aspartame has been linked with problems in many systems in the body. It is often found in foods described as 'low sugar', 'sugar free', or 'diet'.

Junk food

It is a fact that chemically 'enhanced' foods sap our energy resources. The body uses a great deal of energy in the digestion, absorption, cleansing and elimination of foods. It uses far more energy in striving to metabolize low-quality foods, which, unfortunately, hold little nutritional value.

In fibromyalgia particularly, the body is unable to find sufficient energy to complete the digestive process efficiently. As a result, toxins and debris can be stored in the body. Unfortunately, toxic build-up affects every part of the body, from the neurons of the brain to the arteries, kidneys and liver.

Water

There is much ongoing discussion as to the suitability of tap water for human consumption. Water in the UK is thought to be superior to that of a number of other countries. However, it is still laden with toxic chemicals and inorganic salts that are detrimental to those with fibromyalgia.

In areas of 'hard' water, where rainwater has run through limestone (containing sodium salts and calcium salts), our tap water has a high mineral content, particularly of mineral salts. Drinking such water can result in fluid retention and a concentration of salts in our tissues. Ultimately, it can even lead to high blood pressure and hardening of the arteries. 'Soft' water, on the other hand, is usually filtered through sandstone and peat, which removes many of the impurities. This is better, until chemicals are added, such as chlorine and, in some areas, fluoride.

Our water is taken from the following sources:

- **Reservoirs** The aforementioned chemicals are added to this surface water.

- **Deep artesian wells** The purest source of water, artesian water is added to reservoirs.
- **Groundwater** A high content of suspended matter and dissolved acids give groundwater its brown colour. Aluminium sulphate is added as a coagulant, then chemical polyelectrolytes are put in to further settle the coagulated waste. Although this water is then passed through sand filters to remove the settled particles, some of the chemicals remain in the water, which is then added to reservoir water.

As a result of the processes to which water is submitted, it can end up being saturated with inappropriate mineral salts and added chemicals. Other pollutants that often seep in then compound the situation. Your local water authority will provide on request a breakdown of the water content in your postal area.

As tap water is of some detriment to people with fibromyalgia, I recommend that purified water be used. The following types of water are recommended.

- **Distilled water** Formed by boiling water and condensing the steam, distilled water is very pure. It successfully leaches excessive minerals and other salts from the body, but must only be used for periods of up to six months or else essential minerals are at risk of being removed as well. For maximum effect, not more than one of six or eight small glasses of distilled water must be drunk every hour. The results can be spectacular when used as an adjunct to the detoxification diet. However, retailers of distilled water can be hard to locate. (The detoxification programme is discussed in Chapter 7.)
- **Filtered water** Although distilled water has superior effects to filtered water during the detoxification diet, filtered water should be used to maintain your health. Water filters on the market vary from simple carbon filters to carbon filters with silver mesh components that even destroy bacteria. There are also reverse osmosis filters and these produce very clean water while still retaining some of the precious trace minerals. It must be said, however, that the individual effectiveness at removing pollutants is proportionate to their cost. Do not let this put you off, though. An inexpensive carbon filter is far better than no filter at all. (See the Useful addresses section at

the back of the book for details of a recommended water filter manufacturer.)

Note that distilled or filtered water should also be used to wash foods and make drinks.

Refined white flours

Refined wheat flour is generally known to us as plain flour, but can also be called bread flour or pastry flour. In this instance, 'refined' means that the husks have been removed and the remaining powder bleached. This results in the loss of its nutritional value – vitamins, minerals, protein and the fibre content all being removed by these processes. Only carbohydrates and calories remain.

Fortified flours have, as the name implies, had many of their nutrients replaced. However, vitamin B6 and folacin are not put back. Also, of the nine minerals initially removed, only three – iron, calcium and phosphorus – are returned. To compound the situation, many of the replaced processed nutrients have a very slow absorption rate when consumed. So, all in all, refined flours have little nutritional value.

Refined cornflour, or cornmeal, undergoes a less radical refinement process, so loses less of its nutritional content. The oils within the corn can turn rancid, however, if the 'meal' is not freshly ground.

Healthy flour substitutes include wholemeal, spelt, quinoa, oat, maize, brown rice, rye, barley, potato and rice flours, all of which are rich in nutrients. Healthfood shops stock healthy bread mixes that are easy to prepare and nutritious.

Toxic chemicals

Interestingly, apart from a few exceptions, it is no coincidence that in countries with little industrial power and where fresh food is eaten straight from the land, few people suffer chemical sensitivities, food intolerances and/or allergies.

Perhaps the most commonly contracted sensitivity is to 'organophosphates', which are now widely used in farming throughout the Western world.

Organophosphates

Organophosphates (known as OPs) are extremely toxic chemicals used in crop production as a matter of course. It may surprise you to know that every system in the body can be adversely affected by OPs – particularly the immune system, which gives us antibody protection against disease; the central nervous system, which is the nerve processing centre; and the endocrine system, which regulates hormone levels. All the aforementioned systems function abnormally in fibromyalgia.

Typical symptoms of OP poisoning include mental and physical fatigue, poor muscle stamina, muscle pain, drug intolerance, irritable bowel syndrome, sweating, low body temperature, numb patches, muscle twitching, clumsiness, mood swings, irritability, poor short-term memory and poor concentration. Many people with fibromyalgia display all these symptoms.

Evidence of OP poisoning can be found in the following ways.

- **Immune system** Tests can show low levels of B cells, abnormal T suppressor/helper lymphocyte ratios, raised C reactive protein and other abnormalities.
- **Hormones** Tests can show that the pituitary gland is suppressed. This will promote borderline thyroid activity, mild adrenal stress, low levels of sex hormones and low melatonin levels. As a result, the individual will suffer lethargy, weight gain, dry hair and skin, anxiety, low sex drive and sleep difficulties.
- **Cognitive function** Psychometric tests can show impairment of short-term memory, the processing of information, concentration and the ability to learn.
- **Autonomic nervous system** Nerve conduction testing can show abnormalities in many automatic functions. These include body temperature, sweating, gut function, heart and respiratory rate, blood pressure and so on.
- **Liver function** Tests can show whether liver enzyme levels are slightly raised.
- **Blood count** Tests can show low white cell count.
- **Trace element levels** Tests can show deficiencies of the mineral magnesium.
- **Vitamins** Tests can show deficiencies of the B vitamins.

Scary, isn't it? However, if you have fibromyalgia you can begin to eradicate these effects by consuming organically grown produce. The body can be aided in the detoxification of OPs by taking magnesium, selenium and vitamin B12 supplements (see Chapter 5 for more information on the supplements useful in treating fibromyalgia).

Chemical sensitivities

People who are sensitive to OPs may gradually become sensitive to other chemicals. This is known as the 'spreading phenomenon'. Multiple chemical sensitivities – sometimes referred to as allergies – are common in fibromyalgia, sufferers often becoming sensitive to all manner of man-made products. They can react adversely to perfumes, cigarette smoke, alcohol, pesticides, artificial fertilizers, petrochemical fumes, glue, varnish, aerosol sprays, some carpets, some cosmetics, some household cleaners, some paints, etc.

Sensitization to chronic chemical exposure is now well documented. Mechanics can become sensitized to petrol fumes, painters to paint, printers to ink, and so on. Maybe we should all take a closer look at our immediate environments.

The body's tolerance of chemicals can be raised, however, by following the fibromyalgia healing diet, taking plenty of rest and relaxation and adhering to a regular, gentle exercise regime.

Heavy metals

You may be surprised to learn that our bodies commonly absorb heavy metals that are toxic to our systems. The following are the chief culprits.

Aluminium

Believed to be highly implicated in the evolution and persistence of fibromyalgia, high levels of aluminium are harmful to the central nervous system.

Sources of aluminium poisoning may be foil, cookware, containers and underarm deodorants. This metal can also be found in coffee, bleached white flour and antacid medications.

Interestingly, experts are now of the opinion that magnesium and calcium deficiencies increase the toxic effects of ingested aluminium.

Mercury

Those of us with amalgam tooth fillings are ingesting minute amounts of mercury vapour every day – and mercury is the second most toxic heavy metal in the world. The leaked mercury vapour confuses the immune system into attacking the body's own tissues, including the muscles, tendons and ligaments. For this reason, mercury fillings are thought to be implicated in the onset of fibromyalgia.

As a result of mercury intake, the immune system also sets up antibodies against certain foods, thus causing the many food intolerances we see in fibromyalgia. Synthetic white fillings may be a safe alternative.

Lead

Ingestion of this metal is known to cause neurological and psychological disturbance. Some old houses still have lead piping, through which the drinking water is carried, while others have copper piping fused together with lead-based solder. The use of a water filter is highly recommended in such cases, although, obviously, to have the piping replaced by modern copper or synthetic piping is the ideal.

I would like to reinforce my earlier point that fruits and vegetables should be washed in filtered water before use to help remove unwanted substances. A tablespoonful of vinegar may be added to the water to aid this process.

Cadmium

High carbohydrate consumption is linked with high cadmium levels in the body. Cigarette smoking is another cause of cadmium build-up – cadmium being mainly absorbed via the lungs. This metal is known to be damaging to the kidneys and lungs. It can, however, be gradually removed by a detoxification diet, followed by good nutrition.

7

On your way to better health – the detoxification programme

Large amounts of pesticides, food additives and preservatives, toxic chemicals, heavy metals and stimulants can be stored in our organs and tissues, perpetuating fibromyalgia and laying us open to further disease. Although only small amounts of pollutants are ingested each day, over many years – even decades – it can result in toxic overload, some experts estimating that certain adults carry kilos of toxic byproducts and waste. These experts believe that we consume approximately 3.75 litres (1 gallon) of pesticides (found on fresh foods) and 5 kg (11¼ lbs) of chemical food additives a year.

The detoxification process gives the body a well-earned rest, allowing it to concentrate on eliminating toxins and regenerating damaged tissues. Detoxification ensures that toxic byproducts and waste are pulled from the cells into the bloodstream, from where they reach the liver and kidneys, the organs of detoxification. These two organs then work to eliminate the toxins from the body.

Cleansing will only occur, however, if we provide our bodies with cleansing fuel. Fruits, vegetables, juices and water are perfect for this process as they require minimal digestion. The energy saved is then utilized for the elimination of toxins and debris. Secondary to these are whole grains and cereals, oils, nuts, seeds, herbs and spices. They are not only useful in detoxification but also contain important nutrients and use minimum energy during their digestion and elimination.

Nutritionists recommend a 21-day detoxification programme for people with fibromyalgia, after which an improved diet, the type of which is described in this book, should be followed. However, I recommend that you read this chapter before commencing the detoxification programme.

Retraining your palate

The fibromyalgia healing diet and detoxification programme require that you retrain your palate to accept foods in their more natural form. People who have eaten a lot of sugar, salt and saturated fats (those that are solid at room temperature) have come to expect those particular tastes. I recommend, therefore, that, before embarking on the detoxification programme, you cut back gradually on the amounts of sugar, salt and fat you consume. At the same time, try to slowly replace products made from white refined flour with products made from wholegrain flours and use only wholegrain flours in cooking and baking.

The following steps are recommended as part of such a gradual change.

- Eat one biscuit instead of two and slice yourself a smaller piece of cake prior to cutting out or minimizing foods made with butter, sugar and white refined flour.
- To get extra vitamins and minerals, add chopped, cooked vegetables to a tin of soup before cutting out or minimizing use of tinned products.
- Reduce your intake of caffeine products very gradually. Withdrawing too fast may cause fatigue and headaches. If possible, remove caffeine from your diet before commencing the detoxification programme.
- Get into the habit of snacking on a variety of nuts, such as almonds, cashews, Brazils and pecans, dried fruit, such as raisins, dates and apricots, and seeds, such as pumpkin, sesame, sunflower and linseeds.
- Select a salad or vegetables instead of chips when eating out.
- Get into the habit of drinking fruit juice instead of carbonated drinks, which affect carbon levels within the body. Fruit juices generally satisfy a sweet tooth and can be diluted with water so they go further.
- Slowly increase the number and variety of fruits and vegetables you use.
- Gradually reduce the amount of salt you add to your food and in cooking, using rock or sea salt in place of table salt.
- If you find you are craving sugar, remember that the lift it offers will be very temporary – the next effect being a plummet into a

low mood. Staving off hunger with fruit (fresh and dried), nuts and seeds is not only a far healthier choice, it also stabilizes blood-sugar levels, helping to ward off the low mood. (See the Useful addresses section at the back of this book for details of a product that helps diminish cravings for foods and cigarettes.)

• Wash fruit and vegetables thoroughly before use, adding a little vinegar to the distilled or filtered water you use. If you do buy produce that is not organically grown, remember that it will probably have been sprayed with pesticides.

I will just add that, in adulthood, we often do things we do not particularly enjoy. We do them, however, because it is the right thing to do. Cutting down on pleasant foods can be difficult, but our cravings for these foods really can disappear, given a little time and determination.

I must mention also that the people who follow this diet generally admit to finding it enjoyable after the first few weeks. There is no need to become obsessive about it, though! Any improvement in your diet will benefit your condition.

The detoxification superfoods

Here you will find lists of the foods that are known to be powerful detoxifiers. If possible, your detoxification programme should mainly consist of the following.

Fruit

Try to make fruit a staple of your detoxification programme. Not only is it packed with vitamins, minerals, amino acids and enzymes, but its high fibre content means that it is a perfect internal cleanser, too. The fibre binds with toxins and the water content of fruit helps to flush them out. In addition, the pectin in fruit is known to bind with certain heavy metals, helping to carry them from the body.

• **Lemons** During detoxification, try to start your day with a glass of hot water with freshly squeezed lemon juice. As well as providing vitamin C, lemon juice stimulates the liver and gallbladder. It is a powerful cleanser and antiseptic.

• **Apples** Containing malic and tartaric acid, apples boost digestion and aid the removal of impurities from the liver. Their high fibre and pectin content also ensure that they help to eliminate toxins and purify the system. Apples are rich in vitamin C and beta-carotene.

- **Oranges** This fruit stimulates digestion and, as well as containing high levels of vitamin C and other nutrients, is a powerful antioxidant.
- **Grapefruit** Grapefruit is not only high in vitamin C, beta-carotene, calcium, phosphorus and potassium but also stimulates digestion.
- **Pears** Because of their high water content, pears are a diuretic, stimulating the removal of excess water from the body. They contain vitamin C, fibre, potassium and pectin.
- **Bananas** Containing fibre, vitamins and potassium, bananas provide plenty of energy, making them useful during detoxification.
- **Grapes** This fruit is one of the most effective detoxifiers. Grapes are beneficial, too, for disorders of the liver, kidneys, digestion and skin. As they are often sprayed liberally with pesticides, though, it is important to wash them thoroughly or buy organic ones.
- **Melons** Because of their high water content, melons are diuretics, aiding the removal of any excess fluid from the body. They contain vitamin C and beta-carotene.
- **Pineapples** This fruit contains bromelain – an antibacterial agent that aids the digestion of protein. It also has anti-inflammatory properties.
- **Cherries** Containing vitamin C, B vitamins and potassium, cherries assist the removal of toxins from the liver, kidneys and digestive system. The darker the cherry, the more effective it will be.
- **Mangoes** Rich in vitamin C, beta-carotene and potassium, mangoes can cleanse the blood. For this reason, they are of great benefit during the detoxification programme.

As dried fruit is a good source of nutrients, it is also a useful detoxifier. Fruit juices have great benefits, too, as they are so easy to digest. In addition, they help to speed up the metabolism, improve energy levels and stimulate the cleansing process.

Vegetables

Like fruit, vegetables should be a mainstay of a detoxification programme. Vegetables are full of vitamins, minerals, bioflavonoids and plant nutrients (phytochemicals). They also exert a calming effect on the body.

- **Carrots** These vegetables are believed to cleanse, nourish and stimulate the whole body, particularly the kidneys, liver and digestive system. Fresh carrot juice offers the best benefits.
- **Onions, garlic and leeks** With their excellent antiviral and antibacterial nutrients, these vegetables are said to cleanse the whole system. Garlic boosts the immune system and has anti-inflammatory properties.
- **Broccoli, cabbage, cauliflower, Brussels sprouts, watercress and swede** Members of the 'cruciferous' family, these vegetables not only stimulate the liver but also stimulate the body's enzyme defences, thereby playing a vital role in fighting disease.
- **Spinach** This vegetable is rich in beta-carotene and vitamin C. It also contains many more important antioxidant nutrients and is an excellent aid to detoxification.
- **Tomatoes** Containing many vital nutrients, tomatoes are said to stimulate the liver and so aid the removal of toxins.
- **Celery** This vegetable helps to remove excess fluid from the body.
- **Cucumber** Also a diuretic, cucumber aids digestion and relaxes the system.
- **Lettuce** Containing vitamin C, beta-carotene, folate and iron, lettuce has calming, sedative properties. The darker the leaf, the more nutritious it is.

Grains

Because whole grains and cereals are excellent sources of protein, complex carbohydrates, fibre, vitamins and minerals, they play a vital role in a detoxification programme. Look for grains that are largely unprocessed as their high fibre content will speed up the passage of food through the bowel. Examples are brown rice, couscous, millet, barley, bulgar wheat, whole wheat, oats, barley, rye, maize, spelt, quinoa and buckwheat.

Beans and pulses

Similarly, the high fibre content of beans and pulses such as lentils, soya beans, chickpeas and dried peas makes them an important component of the detoxification programme. They are also highly nutritious.

If you are unable to find organic beans that are tinned in water, dried beans are a good alternative. However, most dried beans require soaking for at least eight hours prior to cooking. The preparation instructions should then be carefully followed, especially for kidney beans as otherwise they can be harmful.

Nuts and seeds

Nuts and seeds support the immune system during the detoxification process. They are also excellent sources of nutrients and oils. However, as they are high in fat, they should be eaten in moderation. Salted, coated nuts should be avoided, though.

Oils and vinegars

Although unsaturated oils (fat) – those that are liquid at room temperature – are an important part of a detoxification programme, saturated fat should be avoided. Oils such as extra virgin olive oil and cold-pressed oils such as safflower, sunflower and rapeseed oils provide essential fatty acids as well as vitamin E.

Organic apple cider vinegar stimulates digestion and has many health-giving properties. Other vinegars are not recommended as they contain acetic acid, which hinders digestion.

Coconut oil or snake oil?

Coconut oil has been claimed as a wonder food for everything from weight loss to chronic fatigue syndrome, thyroid disease and Alzheimer's. Anecdotal evidence suggests that some people may find virgin coconut oil helpful in fibromyalgia, the main results being a reduction in pain and an increase in energy. However, at the time of writing, clinical research into coconut oil for fibromyalgia is in its infancy, and there's no scientific evidence that it helps in fibromyalgia, or that it provides any of the many other health benefits claimed for it.

Reports on the internet suggest that some people are taking three to four tablespoons of virgin coconut oil a day to try to improve their fibromyalgia symptoms. Given that one table-spoon of coconut oil contains about 117 calories and 12 grams of saturated fat, it might be better to start small, with a teaspoon or two a day, and then maybe build up to slightly higher doses if you do experience any benefits. The taste and texture can be a problem for some people but it can be enjoyed in smoothies – or use it instead of your other cooking oils, rather than in addition to them.

The energy boost is thought to be due to the fact that coconut oil goes straight to the liver where it is used directly by the body for energy. Most saturated fats contain long-chain fatty acids, which are metabolized via the stomach, to be stored by the body as fat deposits. Coconut oil, however, contains medium-chain fatty acids, which are not digested and laid down as fat in the normal way, but are sent direct to the liver where they are rapidly digested and metabolized to ketone bodies to be used instantly as energy.

Some research has also linked medium-chain fats to increased metabolism in brain cells. Anecdotal evidence and some very pre-liminary research suggests that energy or ketones made in the liver in this way might be effective in boosting the brain in Alzheimer's disease – a possibility for helping with 'fibro fog'? More research is needed, though.

Based on the fact that the body 'combusts' rather than 'absorbs' medium-chain oils, researchers led by Peter Jones, Professor of Dietetics and Nutrition at McGill University, Quebec, Canada, designed a weight-loss cooking oil using coconut and other trop-ical oils. Two studies on the new blend of oil, published in the *International Journal of Obesity*, showed that men lost an average of a pound a month – though women did not experience any notice-able weight loss. However, in both men and women, metabolism was boosted, and cholesterol levels were lowered by an impressive 13 per cent. There was also some encouraging data suggesting that medium-chain oils might help reduce appetite. However, coconut oil played a very small part in the experiment – it made up just six per cent of the study's oil blend.

Cider vinegar

Cider vinegar, purported to be rich in minerals and other nutri-ents, is an ancient remedy for arthritic and many other conditions including swelling or oedema, excess weight, acne and other skin conditions, headaches, cramps, chronic fatigue and sinus troubles. It is believed to cleanse the body, boost metabolism and fight infection. In fibromyalgia, arthritis and gout, cider vinegar is said to help balance the body's pH so that it remains in a slightly alkaline state, thus eliminating acidosis which can cause painful muscle spasms and other symptoms.

Anecdotal reports suggest that cider vinegar may help alleviate symptoms in some people with fibromyalgia, though others find it difficult to tolerate as it appears to irritate the stomach. Try it in small amounts to start with – a teaspoon a day, plus a teaspoon of honey, mixed in warm water; or add to salad dressing in the normal way. Increase the dose in line with your tolerance, aiming for two teaspoons in water with each meal, but do desist if you experience heartburn or other indigestion symptoms. Ensure the cider vinegar is organic, not the standard supermarket brand (e.g. Aspall Organic Cyder Vinegar). For more information, see *Cider Vinegar* by Margaret Hills (Sheldon Press, new edition 2014).

Herbs

Valued for their therapeutic qualities, herbs can be useful during a detoxification programme. The most beneficial include milk thistle, echinacea, ginger root, gotu kola, goldenseal and dandelion leaf and root. Herbal tea infusions are nourishing and cleansing, too.

Spices

Spices have a cleansing, antiseptic effect on the body. Fresh ginger root is a powerful healing spice, as are cardamom, cinnamon, coriander, turmeric, nutmeg and fenugreek.

Turmeric

Turmeric, the pungent yellow spice used in Indian and Asian cooking, is believed to relieve joint pain, stiffness and muscle spasms. It's thought that curcumin, the active ingredient in turmeric, has anti-inflammatory properties, though it's still unclear whether fibromyalgia is in fact an inflammatory condition. A 2012 preliminary study of patients with rheumatoid arthritis found that curcumin improved symptoms of joint swelling and tenderness, although more research is needed.

It's sometimes recommended that you take turmeric with ginger (a pleasant and well-established combination in a curry). Don't go overboard though – too much turmeric can cause side effects such as indigestion, dizziness, diarrhoea or nausea. If you're considering curcumin supplements (rather than routine use of the turmeric spice powder in cooking), be careful not to exceed the recommended dose. Turmeric supplements are also not recommended for pregnant and breastfeeding women, as they can stimulate the uterus and cause bleeding. You should also avoid supplements if you have gall bladder problems, are facing surgery, or are taking anti-coagulant or diabetic medication.

Guaifenesin

Guaifenesin, the over-the-counter cough and cold preparation, is a controversial treatment for fibromyalgia. A study by the world-renowned rheumatologist Dr Robert Bennett, Professor of Medicine and Nursing at Oregon Health and Science University, failed to show that it is effective. The research found that there was no real difference between the group taking a placebo and the group taking guaifenesin. It was concluded that any improvements were due to the 'placebo effect', where the person's belief in a medication is so strong they actually do feel better for a while, although it's also been noted that guaifenesin can cause side effects including headaches and dizziness.

The theory is that guaifenesin works to remove excess phosphate in our cells, which disrupts muscle function in fibromyalgia, causing spasm and pain. It's also speculated that any effect may be due to guaifenesin's action as a muscle relaxant. Dr R. Paul St Amand, who has been using guaifenesin for the treatment of fibromyalgia since the1990s, professes to have seen great success in his patients. However, he stresses that for guaifenesin to be effective, patients must reduce their intake of salicylates, found in aspirin and many foodstuffs. Avoiding salicylates in itself may improve fibromyalgia, especially if you suspect you may have an allergy to them – an estimated 70 per cent of those with IBS are sensitive to salicylates (IBS is found in approximately 15 per cent of the general population, but in

Table 7.1 Foods to avoid if you are sensitive to salicylates

Foods to avoid or eat only in small quantities	
Dried fruits	Endives
Berry fruits	Olives
Oranges	Grapes
Apricots	Almonds
Pineapples	Liquorice
Cucumbers	Peppermints
Gherkins	Honey
Tomato sauce	Worcestershire sauce
Tea	Many spices

up to 70 per cent of people with fibromyalgia). Salicylate sensitivity is also thought to play a part in more than 20 per cent of asthma cases.

Salicylates are natural chemicals found in some fresh produce foods, and also manufactured in certain foods. They may also feature in beauty products. If you suspect you are sensitive to salicylates, try avoiding or limiting the foods in Table 7.1 for two to four weeks. This should be enough to tell if excluding them makes a difference to your fibromyalgia.

Meat and dairy products

Because animal protein foods, such as meat and dairy products, put a strain on kidney function, they should, ideally, be avoided during the detoxification programme. These organs will be working flat out to eliminate toxins.

Dairy products are mucus-forming, too, and mucus will not only be present in the nasal and respiratory passages, it can also lurk in virtually every part of the body. In the bowel, mucus slows the transport of waste material, hampering the elimination of toxins and debris. Alternative foods include soya milk, rice milk, goats' milk and cheese, and tofu yogurts. The only divergence during detoxification should be butter, which must be spread very thinly on your wholemeal breads and rye crispbreads, and natural live yogurt can be eaten, too.

Natural live yogurt

Eating a helping of natural live yogurt every day will improve the condition of your gut flora during detoxification. Natural live yogurt contains beneficial bacteria that rebalance the gut flora.

Keeping a diary

Keeping a food intake diary is an excellent way to monitor your progress. Seeing for yourself where you are making mistakes will ensure a smoother changeover to healthier eating.

Goals

It is a good idea to set goals at the start of the diary. For example, you may want to make a goal of eating two types of vegetables every day. Without the diary, you may assume you have done badly, but, on reading your entries, you may see that you have actually eaten two types of vegetables three or four times a week. That is a good starting point. Now you can focus on slowly increasing that amount. (Remember that it is important to become accustomed to the new foods in your diet before commencing the detoxification programme.)

Here are some examples of goals towards maximum healing:

- eat two to three types of vegetables every day;
- eat two to three portions of fruit every day;
- cut out caffeine – coffee, chocolate, cola drinks, cocoa;
- cut out junk food;
- cut out table sugar and other sugar-containing products, such as cakes, sweets, biscuits, sugar-coated cereals and so on;
- cut out saturated fats;
- cut out refined white flour;
- eat only 'whole' foods – whole wheat, corn, barley, brown rice and so on;
- drink eight to ten glasses of clean water daily, including that in fruit juices and herbal teas;
- cut out or minimize table salt sprinkled on food, using small amounts of sea or rock salt instead;
- minimize the amount of salt added to cooking and baking;
- reduce your intake of meat and dairy products to a minimum,

making sure to spread butter thinly (meat and dairy products should, ideally, be avoided for the duration of the detoxification programme);
- minimize alcohol consumption;
- eat nuts, seeds and/or dried fruit as snacks once or twice a day;
- cut out artificial sweeteners;
- always check food labels for additives, preservatives and so on;
- buy only organically grown produce;
- use vegetable, corn or olive oil in cooking and dressings – extra virgin olive oil is best;
- cut out fried foods.

Note that if you are unable to entirely eliminate certain foods, you should not feel discouraged. Cutting down your intake will reduce the strain on your digestive system and detoxification organs, making a difference to your health.

A symptom column

It is also important to include a symptom column at the end of each week. It should include average energy levels, pain levels, headaches/migraines, muscle cramps, stiffness, aching joints, mood, sleep quality, stomach problems, cold hands and feet, general tiredness, concentration, short-term memory and stress levels. Each entry should be marked on a scale of one to ten, with the lowest numbers being the least intensity and higher numbers being greater intensity. This should show improvements that may otherwise be overlooked.

Weight matters

It is no wonder that many people with fibromyalgia are overweight. Fibromyalgia demands that we are fairly inactive, cell energy production is limited and our metabolisms are sluggish.

As you will know, being overweight can be damaging to health. Its related conditions include high blood pressure, heart disease, diabetes, chronic anxiety and depression. However, it is not wise to lose weight by following either a crash diet or a diet that limits certain foods. Such diets almost certainly result in substantial weight loss in the early weeks, but the long-term result is actually weight gain. This occurs because the body goes into starvation mode, storing energy as fat in the cell pockets. Unfortunately, when the diet peters out, the weight piles on.

However, a happy side-effect of a detoxification programme, followed by a good-quality diet, is weight loss in people who were overweight. Furthermore, because the foods used are low in calories, any excess fat comes away – and with it all the toxins stored there!

Study after study has pinpointed the close link between weight gain and fibromyalgia, although it's a bit of a chicken-and-egg situation. While being overweight or obese is not thought in itself to cause fibromyalgia, it certainly appears to aggravate symptoms. It may also be a factor in the link between fibromyalgia and diabetes.

One study also found that more gain equals more pain. That is, the greater the weight increase, the more severe the symptoms are likely to be, such as chronic pain, fatigue, sleep disturbance and mood disorders. The study, published in the journal *Arthritis Care & Research* in 2012, looked at 888 adults with fibromyalgia. Study co-author Dr Terry Oh, assistant professor of physical medicine and rehabilitation at the Mayo Clinic, in Rochester, Minnesota, found that severely obese patients had more tender points and worse physical functioning than the non-obese and less obese.

It's probably no news to you that fibromyalgia can be disabling as well as debilitating. A 2011 study by University of Utah researchers, reported in the *Journal of Pain*, found a close association between obesity and disability in people with fibromyalgia. In the study, 215 people with fibromyalgia were assessed to see if obesity added to the disease and disability burden of the condition. As with previous studies, obesity was found to be common – half the people in the study sample were obese and an additional 30 per cent were overweight. Obese patients had increased pain sensitivity, especially in lower body areas, and reduced flexibility and strength in the lower body. They also experienced more disturbed and restless sleep. This was consistent with previous findings.

There are several reasons why you might gain weight with fibromyalgia. When it hurts to move, sadly you're much less likely to exercise. Tiredness and sleep deprivation also militate against exercise. Metabolic factors, thyroid disease and depression are also possible factors, and certain medicines such as some antidepressants and anti-epileptic drugs also cause weight gain as a side effect. However, some critics have suggested that these studies be viewed more in context, bearing in mind that the prevalence of obesity has risen greatly in the normal population.

It's less clear whether losing weight banishes fibromyalgia – though it certainly helps. A 2005 study at the State University of New York, Albany, looked at women with fibromyalgia who did a 20-week weight-loss programme. The women lost an average of 9 lbs with corresponding improvements in pain, body satisfaction and quality of life.

If you are concerned about your weight, you might find it helpful to track it with an online tool such as SparkPeople (<www.sparkpeople.com>) or MyFitnessPal (<www.myfitnesspal.com>).

A healing crisis

It is not all roses, however. A detoxification diet releases toxins and debris into the bloodstream, where they circulate until reaching the liver and kidneys. These organs then neutralize the toxins and prepare them for elimination. When the quantity of toxins exceeds the body's ability to remove them, though, detoxification reactions can occur. Toxins lingering in the bloodstream can cause lethargy, headaches and occasionally even diarrhoea.

The good news is that the feeling of unwellness lasts for only a few days. Please do not let these possible side-effects demotivate you for the ill feeling is a positive indication that the toxins are in the process of being removed. It is a sure sign that you are on your way to improved health. I must add that many people suffer no adverse reactions whatsoever.

Purified water

During a detoxification programme, distilled water is by far the most beneficial (see Chapter 6). It not only has cleansing properties but is also capable of drawing heavy metals, salts and other debris from the tissues. Drinking eight to ten glasses of distilled water daily will considerably reduce detoxifying symptoms. After the detoxification programme has been completed, you can return to filtered water.

If you are not able to obtain distilled water for your detoxification programme, filtered water is an acceptable alternative. I would highly recommend that filtered water then be drunk for the rest of your life. However, if filtered water is not available, mineral water should be used. It is not the best choice, as it does not draw detrimental salts and so on from the tissues effectively, but is superior to tap water. Another method of 'cleaning' your drinking water is to allow a jugful to stand in the freezer for a few hours before use. Remember to wash your fruit and vegetables in distilled or filtered or mineral water with a tablespoonful of vinegar added before eating or cooking.

Ready to go!

Before getting started on the 21-day detoxification programme, it is advisable to consciously tell yourself you are making an important lifestyle decision – to eat better. Remember that, as a result, your health will improve, the possibility of future illness will be reduced and you can look forward to a longer life!

The following guidelines should help you on your way to improved health:

- make optimum nutrition a goal – remind yourself of the importance of this goal to your health;
- make a conscious effort to change past bad eating behaviour;
- be organized – plan meals in advance;
- eat three to five portions of fruit every day;
- eat three to five portions of vegetables every day, trying to occasionally eat raw vegetables, such as grated carrots with a salad;
- eat whole grains and cereals, nuts, beans, pulses, seeds, herbs, spices and the recommended oils;
- remember that fat must not be eliminated – consumption of unsaturated fat, which is oils that are liquid at room temperature, is essential for improved health;
- avoid skipping meals, particularly breakfast;
- boil, bake and steam your foods – eggs should be soft-boiled or poached;
- avoid overeating;
- do not ever go hungry;
- drink eight to ten glasses of water a day, including that in fruit and vegetable drinks and herbal teas;

- if possible, try to keep busy to prevent boredom – this will help with any inclination you may feel towards eating to occupy time;
- avoid weighing and measuring yourself on a regular basis – instead, feel the benefit in the fit of your clothing;
- keep alcohol consumption very low, remembering that red wine is the best choice when you do have the odd drink;
- practise pain and stress management – daily deep breathing and relaxation exercises should cut stress levels and try to deal with negative thinking and irrational feelings by forward planning, being realistic and speaking openly of your limitations to others (my previous book, *Living with Fibromyalgia* (third edition, Sheldon Press, 2014) tackles pain and stress management in detail);
- follow a daily exercise programme, expanding your routine and increasing the number of repetitions as you grow stronger, and ensure that you perform an aerobic activity – an exercise that makes you a little out of breath – at least once every other day;
- focus on getting well.

Your 21-day detoxification programme

Just to reiterate, it is advisable to gradually accustom yourself to the different foods in your new diet. Giving yourself at least one month where you gradually introduce more and more of the recommended foods means that it is not such a shock to the system. This allows you time to get used to the tastes of newly introduced foods.

After a month – or longer if you wish – you can begin the 21-day detoxification programme in earnest. The following are important points to remember:

- try to start your day with a glass of hot water with some freshly squeezed lemon juice added;
- eat a healthy breakfast, lunch and evening meal, but do not pile up the plate – if possible, consume 25 per cent of your daily intake at breakfast, 50 per cent at lunch and 25 per cent in the evening, but, if you cannot manage this, do not worry, just make sure you do not eat too much towards the end of the day;
- eat regular snacks of fresh fruit, dried fruit, raw vegetables, nuts, seeds, crispbreads and so on (nuts and seeds – particularly cashew

and pecan nuts, linseeds, sesame seeds and sunflower seeds – are excellent sources of essential oils and other important nutrients);

- increase your consumption of raw fruits, nuts, seeds and vegetables to at least 50 per cent of your diet – 'fruit and vegetables' should include apples, grapefruit, oranges, grapes, cherries, pineapple, avocados, melons, spinach, broccoli, Brussels sprouts, cabbage, lettuce, cucumber, radishes, onions, carrots and capsicum peppers;
- try to cut out all dairy products except natural live yogurt and butter, remembering to use only a small amount of the latter;
- eat whole grains and cereals, such as whole wheat, oats, barley, maize, couscous, millet, spelt and brown rice;
- eat beans, peas, pulses, lentils, herbs and spices;
- use olive, corn, safflower and sunflower oils;
- buy only organically grown produce – the superior taste makes up for the slight difference in cost;
- drink six to eight glasses of distilled or filtered water a day, making this up to the total of eight to ten glasses of liquid recommended by drinking green tea and fruit and vegetable juices;
- have your last snack at least two hours before bedtime – eating a small amount of carbohydrate at the end of the day should encourage sleep;
- strive for a stress-free eating environment – no television or reading while eating;
- take exercise as tolerated (see below);
- take in some fresh air every day (see below);
- get plenty of rest, following a deep breathing and relaxation exercise at least once a day – you may want to use a relaxation CD or download to help you through the process (CDs can be purchased from health shops).

To achieve maximum detoxification, avoid or minimize your intake of the following:

- dairy products and meat – if you are unable to do this, eat only small, lean cuts in portions no larger or thicker than the size of your palm and remember that red meat in particular takes a long time to digest, using energy that could otherwise be utilized in detoxification;
- white refined sugar;

- white refined flour;
- additives and preservatives;
- foods grown using chemicals;
- junk food and salt;
- fried foods;
- caffeine, including coffee, caffeine teas, cola drinks, chocolate and cocoa;
- alcohol;
- tobacco;
- aspartame, saccharine and other refined or artificial sweeteners;
- finally, remember to take your drinks at least half an hour before and half an hour after eating – the greater the gap between eating and drinking, the less likelihood there is of important hydrochloric (stomach) acid being diluted.

Exercise and fresh air

Fundamental to the cleansing process is plenty of gentle, sustained exercise and daily fresh air. Exercise stimulates the lymph glands, which operate as a sewage system and, therefore, are heavily burdened during detoxification. The flow of lymph from the lymph glands is entirely dependent on muscular movement.

I know exercise is difficult for people with fibromyalgia, so keep it gentle. Circling your shoulders backwards and forwards several times a day will be beneficial, as will turning and tilting your head, full body side-dips and side-twists. Walking is good, too. You only need to walk around the house, maybe then climbing the stairs two or three times more than you would normally.

Having said that, fresh air is equally important as toxic gases are dispelled from our bodies via the lungs. The inhalation of clean, fresh oxygen sustains the metabolic reactions within each cell. You do not need to embark on a route march every day, either! A walk around the garden once or twice a day or a short walk along the road should provide sufficient fresh air. If walking is difficult at this early stage, simply wrapping up warmly and standing at the open door or by an open window for a while is far better than nothing. Remember, too, that things will get better!

Nutrition maintenance

You have successfully completed the detoxification programme, so what happens now? Some of you may want to continue in the same vein. In the main, I would advise that you be a little less stringent, but try to eat the foods recommended in this book. Remember that, to continue the healing process, it is important to eat a wide variety of nutritious foods and take the nutritional supplements mentioned in Chapter 5. However, to maintain the detoxification of harmful chemicals and continue strengthening all the systems in the body, the following eating habits should be adhered to in the long term:

- continue to eat three or four small meals a day, remembering not to skip any;
- keep the high fibre content, eating fruits, vegetables, whole grains and cereals;
- have healthy food available at home or work so you can 'snack' whenever you want;
- eat wholemeal breads, pasta and brown rice;
- eat plenty of legumes (peas and beans);
- select low-fat dairy products and keep your intake of them low;
- limit red meats, especially cured and smoked meats, as they are difficult to digest;
- eat white meats, tuna and fish in moderation;
- eat plenty of raw fruit and vegetables, making salads a must;
- consume at least eight glasses of liquid a day, including fruit/vegetable juices and herbal teas.

It is important to remember that if you deviate from your diet – whether during detoxification or afterwards – do not be disheartened. Just return to your healthy foods and forget the slight lapse. There will be times when you prefer to put the diet aside for a while, such as when eating out or during a holiday. This does not mean that you have stopped your healthy diet. Take up where you left off as soon as you can and get back to improving your health.

Suggested menus

The following menus are for use both during and after the detoxification period. Make your helpings of meat and fish very small during detoxification. Note that the cup you should use for the measures given below is a small teacup or American cup measure rather than a mug.

Day 1

Breakfast:	Porridge made with water, raw honey and soya milk
Snack:	⅓ cup pecan nuts
Lunch:	Vegetable Paella (page 115)
Snack:	2 kiwi fruit
Dinner:	Rice Pilaf and Fig Bar (pages 116 and 131)
Snack:	Banana

Day 2

Breakfast:	Grapefruit and 2 slices wholemeal toast
Snack:	⅛ cup sunflower seeds
Lunch:	Artichoke Salad (page 123) and 2 rye crispbreads
Snack:	Raw carrots and celery with fat-free dip
Dinner:	Grilled wild salmon with lemon, potatoes, broccoli, peas
Snack:	⅓ cup cashew nuts

Day 3

Breakfast:	Wedge of canteloupe melon
Snack:	⅓ cup mixed dried fruit and nuts
Lunch:	Tomato and Orange Soup (page 91), wholemeal roll, and 2 Farmhouse Biscuits (page 127)
Snack:	Dried apricots
Dinner:	Home-made vegetable curry and brown rice
Snack:	Apple

Day 4

Breakfast:	Bircher Muesli (page 90) with rice milk
Snack:	Orange
Lunch:	Falafel (similar to a veggie burger and available from healthfood shops), pear
Snack:	2 rye crispbreads with cottage cheese
Dinner:	Chicken Rolls (page 116) with potatoes, green beans and carrots
Snack:	Raw carrots, celery and virtually fat-free dip

Day 5
Breakfast: Fresh fruit salad
Snack: ⅓ cup pecan nuts
Lunch: Modern Ratatouille (page 115) with millet and Lemon
             Mousse (page 124)
Snack: 2 oatcakes (available from healthfood shops)
Dinner: 2 soft-boiled eggs on wholemeal toast and Banana
             Split (page 125)
Snack: Slice Carrot Cake (page 130)

Day 6
Breakfast: Porridge with cracked linseed, molasses and soya milk
Snack: ½ cup dried fruit
Lunch: Baked sweet potato with cottage cheese and pineapple
             and 2 Oatie Bran Fingers (page 131)
Snack: Banana
Dinner: Pasta 'n' Fish (page 118) and an apple
Snack: 1 cup cashew nuts

Day 7
Breakfast: Wholemeal toast with raw honey
Snack: Orange
Lunch: Avocado and Cheese (page 117) with salad and fresh
             fruit salad
Snack: ¼ cup toasted sesame seeds with Kelpamare seasoning
             (available from Bioforce – see the Useful addresses
             section for details)
Dinner: Cajun Fish Fillets and No-fry Chips (pages 109 and
             108)
Snack: 1–2 slice(s) wholemeal bread with peanut butter

As well as being organically grown, the foods used in these menus
should be additive and preservative-free. Do not forget to bring
in the other foods recommended, however, so that, all in all, you
consume a wide variety of foods. The recipes given in Chapter 8
should add further variety.

Part 2
HEALING RECIPES

As already discussed, healthy eating is fundamental to relieving the myriad symptoms of fibromyalgia. It is also the first line of defence against further invasive disease. This part of the book is devoted to recipes using foods that are known to aid the healing process.

Essential basics

Home-made Vegetable Stock

Makes 600 ml (1 pint)

1 tbsp sunflower oil	*4 parsley stalks*
1 potato, chopped	*1 sprig thyme*
1 carrot, chopped	*1 bay leaf*
1 onion, chopped	*pinch freshly ground black pepper*
1 celery stick, chopped	*600 ml (1 pint) filtered water*
2 garlic cloves, peeled	

Heat the sunflower oil in a large saucepan, then add the vegetables. Cover and boil gently for about 10 minutes. Add the herbs, mix and pour the water into the pan. Bring back to the boil, then simmer, partially covered, for 40 minutes. Strain, season with the pepper and use as required. This stock will add flavour to stews and soups or may simply be poured over your steamed vegetables. It can be frozen or stored in a refrigerator for 3–4 days.

Basic Meat Sauce

Serves 8

Submitted by Dorothy Holden

750 g (1½ lbs) lean minced beef or lamb

100 g (4 oz) lean back bacon

2 onions, finely chopped

1 garlic clove, crushed

100 g (4 oz) carrots,finely diced

1 green bell pepper (capsicum), deseeded and finely diced

100 g (4 oz) mushrooms, sliced

2 celery sticks, chopped

500-g (14-oz) tin chopped tomatoes, including juice

75 g (3 oz) tomato purée

pinch sea salt or to taste

pinch freshly ground black pepper

25 g (1 oz) basil, chopped

½ tbsp vegetable stock or Home-made Vegetable Stock (page 85)

½ tbsp cornflour

Place the mince in a large saucepan and sauté (that is, cover and allow to cook in its own steam) over a low heat until it starts to turn brown. Add the bacon, onions, garlic, carrots, pepper (capsicum), mushrooms and celery, stirring all the time. Add the tinned tomatoes, juice and all, and the tomato purée, then season with salt, pepper and basil. Cover and simmer gently for half an hour. Gradually add the stock and flour, stirring well until the desired consistency is achieved. This meat sauce can be frozen when it has cooled.

Savoury Curry Sauce

Serves 4

Cooked red or white meat or frozen seafood can be added to this sauce.

Submitted by Dorothy Holden

2 large onions, finely chopped
4 garlic cloves or to taste,
  crushed
1 tsp coriander, fresh or dried
300 ml (½ pint) filtered water,
  approximately
2 tsp ground cumin
1 tbsp olive oil

1 tsp chilli powder
2 tsp turmeric
1 tsp garam masala
4 tsp paprika
2 tsp dried fenugreek leaves
1 tbsp tomato purée
1 tbsp tomato ketchup
pinch sea salt or to taste

Place the onions and garlic in a frying pan and sauté over a medium heat for 5 minutes. Keeping back a little coriander, mix the spices into a jug of 150 ml (¼ pint) of the water, then add to the pan. Cook for a further 5 minutes, then reduce the heat to a simmer. Add the tomato purée, the ketchup and a little more water, then simmer for about 20 minutes. Keep adding water so it does not become too dry. Add the precooked meat, chicken or frozen seafood, if using, together with a pinch of salt, and heat through, stirring all the time. Serve garnished with the remaining coriander. Remember that meat should only be eaten 2–3 times a week.

Wholemeal Shortcrust Pastry

Makes 450 g (1 lb)

*100 g (4 oz) plain organic
  wholemeal flour
100 g (4 oz) self-raising
  organic wholemeal flour*

*100 g (4 oz) butter
pinch sea salt or to taste
120 ml (4 fl oz) filtered water*

Place the flours, butter and salt in a bowl. Rub the butter into the flour until the mixture resembles fine breadcrumbs. Gradually add the water and mix with a round-ended knife to form a soft dough, then draw together with the fingertips. Leave the dough in the bowl and refrigerate for 5 minutes. Then, roll it out on a floured surface and use as required. Because of its high butter content, try to make this pastry a treat!

Oatmeal Pastry

Makes 450 g (1 lb)

*175 g (6 oz) self-raising
  organic flour
50 g (2 oz) fine oatmeal*

*150 g (5 oz) butter
50 g (2 oz) demerara sugar*

Place the flours and butter in a bowl. Rub the butter in with the fingertips to keep the fat cool. Add the sugar and mix it in with the hands. A little water may be required to bind the mixture to form a dough. Roll it out on a floured surface and use as required. Again, this pastry should be eaten sparingly.

Breakfasts

Breakfast Banana

Serves 2–3

3 small bananas
2 tsp fresh lemon juice
pinch ground cinnamon

50 g (2 oz) uncoated cashew
  nuts, finely chopped or
  ground

Mash 1 banana in a bowl, adding the lemon juice. If required, add a little filtered water to make a smooth paste. Add the cinnamon. Now slice the other bananas and mix into the sauce. Spoon into dessert glasses and garnish with the nuts.

Sweet Potato Beginnings

Serves 3–4

2 sweet potatoes, pierced
2 bananas, sliced
1 apple, peeled, cored and diced
½ tsp ground cinnamon

Bake the sweet potatoes in the microwave on high for 5–7 minutes or until soft. Allow to stand until cool enough to touch, then peel and mash in a bowl. Add the fruit and stir well. Sprinkle with cinnamon and serve hot.

Bircher Muesli

Serves 2

1 apple, coarsely chopped
75 g (3 oz) raisins, washed
1 orange, segmented and
chopped

1 banana, chopped
150 g (5 oz) rolled oats
85–150 ml (3–5 fl oz) soya or
rice milk, to taste

Place all the ingredients in a medium bowl and mix together. Serve.

Soups

Tomato and Orange Soup

Serves 6

225 g (8 oz) potatoes, diced
1 large onion, finely chopped
450 g (1 lb) tomatoes,
   blanched, peeled and
   quartered
600 ml (1 pint) vegetable stock
   or Home-made Vegetable
   Stock (page 85)

zest and juice of 1 orange
½ tsp dried oregano, chopped
pinch sea salt or to taste
pinch freshly ground black
   pepper or to taste
1 orange, quartered
3 slices toasted wholemeal
   bread, diced to make croûtons

Place the potatoes, onion, tomatoes, stock, orange zest and juice, oregano and salt and pepper in a large saucepan. Bring to the boil, cover and simmer gently for 30 minutes. Place in a blender or food processor and blend well, sieving to remove any seeds. Return to the pan and reheat, adding a little more stock if required. Ladle into warmed bowls, garnishing each with a segment of orange and sprinkling the croûtons over.

Gazpacho (Chilled Soup)

Serves 4

450 g (1 lb) tomatoes, roughly
   sliced
1 onion, diced
1 green bell pepper, deseeded
   and diced
1 garlic clove, crushed
1 tbsp olive oil
1 tbsp organic apple cider
   vinegar

juice of 1 lemon
¼ cucumber, diced
pinch sea salt or to taste
pinch freshly ground black
   pepper or to taste
3 slices toasted wholemeal
   bread, diced to make
   croûtons

Place the tomatoes, onion, pepper, garlic, olive oil and vinegar in a blender and combine well. Pour the mixture into a bowl, adding the lemon juice and salt and pepper to taste. Chill in a refrigerator before serving with croûtons.

Carrot Borscht

Serves 4

1 onion, finely chopped
1 large potato, peeled and
    diced
1 tsp olive oil
1 raw beetroot, peeled and
    diced
350 g (12 oz) carrots, peeled
    and diced
1 litre (1¾ pints) vegetable
    stock or Home-made
    Vegetable Stock (page 85)

225 g (8 oz) soft tofu,
    squeezed to remove excess
    liquid (optional)
¼ tsp ground nutmeg
pinch sea salt or to taste
pinch freshly ground black
    pepper or to taste
handful fresh mint, chopped

Place the onion and potato in a large saucepan and sauté very gently in the olive oil for 7–10 minutes, stirring frequently. Add the beetroot and carrots, cover and simmer for another 20 minutes. Pour in the stock and simmer for a further 10 minutes. Add the tofu, if using, then pour the contents of the pan into a blender or food processor. After blending to a smooth consistency, adding the nutmeg and seasoning to taste, ladle the soup into warmed bowls. Garnish with the chopped mint and serve.

Tomato and Lentil Soup

Serves 4

1 large onion, finely chopped
4 tomatoes, skinned and
   quartered
100 g (4 oz) red lentils, rinsed
275 ml (9 fl oz) vegetable
   stock or Home-made
   Vegetable Stock (page 85)

pinch sea salt or to taste
pinch freshly ground black
   pepper or to taste
4 fresh basil leaves, chopped

Place the onion in a large saucepan and sauté in a little water until just softened. Add the tomatoes and lentils, then stir in the stock. Season with salt and pepper. Bring to the boil, cover and simmer gently for 30 minutes or until the lentils are tender. Remove from the heat and pour the mixture into a blender or food processor and process until smooth. Return to the pan and heat through. Ladle into warmed bowls and garnish with the basil.

Cream of Potato Soup

Serves 3

450 g (1 lb) potatoes, peeled
   and diced
1 large onion, finely chopped
2 medium celery sticks, sliced
15 g (½ oz) butter
450 ml (¾ pint) filtered water

pinch sea salt or to taste
pinch freshly ground black
   pepper or to taste
300 ml (½ pint) skimmed milk
2 tbsp chopped fresh parsley

Place the vegetables and the butter in a medium saucepan and add 1 tablespoonful of the water. Sauté very gently for 7–10 minutes. Add the remaining water and season. Bring to the boil, cover and simmer gently for 25 minutes. Pour the soup into a blender or food processor and mix until smooth. Return to the pan and stir in the milk. Bring to the boil once more, stirring well, then cover and simmer for 5 minutes. Ladle into warmed bowls and sprinkle with the parsley.

Cock-a-Leekie Soup

Serves 3

275 g (10 oz) skinless, boned
   chicken, diced
2 tsp olive oil
1 tbsp filtered water
350 g (12 oz) leeks, chopped
   into 2.5-cm (1-in) lengths,
   green parts finely shredded

1.2 litres (2 pints) vegetable
   stock or Home-made
   Vegetable Stock (page 85)
1 bouquet garni
6 prunes, stoned and halved
3 sprigs fresh parsley

Place the chicken, olive oil and water in a medium saucepan and gently sauté until the chicken has browned a little on all sides. Add the white pieces of leek to the pan and continue to cook for a further 5 minutes, until the leeks have softened. Add the stock and bouquet garni. Bring to the boil, then simmer for 30 minutes. Add the green leek pieces and prunes. Simmer for 30 more minutes. Ladle into warmed bowls and garnish with the parsley.

Cabbage and Leek Soup

Serves 6

1.2 litres (2 pints) vegetable
   stock or Home-made
   Vegetable Stock (page 85)
8 leeks, trimmed, washed and
   diced
1.25 kg (2¾ lbs) green or
   Savoy cabbage, stalk and
   outer leaves removed,
   rest chopped into 2-cm
   (¾-in) pieces

1 large onion, finely chopped
pinch sea salt or to taste
pinch freshly ground black
   pepper or to taste
6 slices Granary bread, toasted
   and diced to make croûtons
50 g (2 oz) low-fat organic
   Cheddar cheese, grated
   (optional)

Pour the stock into a large saucepan and bring to the boil. Add the vegetables, then bring back to the boil. Cover and simmer gently for 35–45 minutes, stirring occasionally. Season with the salt and pepper. Ladle into warmed bowls, garnish with the croûtons and sprinkle the cheese over the top, if using.

Main meals

Microwave Chilli con Carne

Serves 4

Submitted by Dorothy Holden

½ × Basic Meat Sauce recipe
(page 86)
1 green bell pepper
(capsicum), deseeded and
thinly sliced
1 tbsp olive oil
1 tbsp red wine vinegar

1 tsp muscovado or demerara
sugar
1–2 tsp chilli powder,
according to taste
1 tbsp ground cumin
1 medium tin red kidney beans,
drained

Reheat the meat sauce from frozen in a microwave by setting it for 10 minutes on 'defrost', then cook on high for 1½ minutes. Allow to stand. Place the pepper in a frying pan and sauté in the olive oil for about 3 minutes or until softened. Stir in the vinegar, sugar, chilli powder and cumin. Mix well. Add to the meat sauce. Add the kidney beans. Cover and microwave on a medium setting for 5 minutes or until heated through.

Microwave Chicken Curry

Serves 4

Submitted by Dorothy Holden

450 g (1 lb) brown rice
1 onion, finely chopped
1 tbsp sunflower oil
1–2 tbsp medium madras curry
    powder or to taste
1 tbsp cornflour
600 ml (1 pint) vegetable stock
    or 1 x Home-made
    Vegetable Stock recipe (page
    85)
1 tsp Worcestershire sauce

2 tsp tomato purée
2 tsp fresh lemon juice
2 tsp mango chutney
1 dessert apple, peeled, cored
    and sliced
50 g (2 oz) sultanas, washed
350 g (12 oz) cooked chicken,
    diced
pinch sea salt or to taste
pinch freshly ground black
    pepper or to taste

Bring a large pan of water to the boil, stir in the rice, cover, reduce the heat and simmer for 30 minutes until tender. Towards the end of the cooking time for the rice, place the onion and sunflower oil in a microwavable dish. Cover and microwave on high for 1½ minutes, then stir. Add the curry powder and cornflour and, stirring well, gradually blend in the stock. Re-cover and microwave on high for 3 minutes or until the sauce has boiled and thickened. Stir, add the Worcestershire sauce, tomato purée, lemon juice, chutney, apple and sultanas and stir again. Cover and microwave on high for 2 minutes. Add the chicken, salt and pepper, then stir and re-cover. Microwave on high for a final 2 minutes or until piping hot. Serve on a ring of brown rice. When cooled, this sauce can be frozen for later use.

Bavarian Beef Stew

Serves 5

450 g (1 lb) lean beef, or
lamb, stewing meat, diced
into 2.5-cm (1-in) pieces
1 tbsp sunflower or other light
oil
1 large onion, finely chopped
¾ tsp caraway seeds
pinch sea salt or to taste
pinch freshly ground black
pepper or to taste

1 bay leaf
200 ml (7 fl oz) cider vinegar
¼ tbsp fructose
½ small head red cabbage, cut
into 4 wedges
200 ml (7 fl oz) vegetable
stock or Home-made
Vegetable Stock (page 85)
50 g (2 oz) crushed gingersnap
biscuits

Place the meat and oil in a heavy-bottomed frying pan and sauté until just turning brown. Remove the meat and sauté the onion in the remaining oil until golden. Return the meat to the pan and add the stock, caraway seeds, salt, pepper and bay leaf. Bring to the boil then cover and simmer gently for 1¼ hours. Add the cider vinegar and fructose, stirring well. Place the cabbage on top of the meat. Cover and simmer for 20 minutes or until the cabbage is tender. Arrange the meat and cabbage on a platter and keep warm. Pour the stock into a small saucepan and add the crushed gingersnaps. Stirring well, cook until thickened. Serve with the meat and vegetables.

Autumn Mashed Potatoes

Serves 6

225 g (8 oz) carrots, thinly
sliced
750 g (1½ lbs) potatoes, peeled
and diced
1 small swede, peeled and
diced
3 parsnips, peeled and diced

50 ml (2 fl oz) skimmed milk
25 g (1 oz) butter
pinch sea salt or to taste
pinch freshly ground black
pepper or to taste
25 g (1 oz) chopped chives
2 sprigs fresh mint (optional)

Place the carrots in a saucepan of boiling water and simmer for 5 minutes. Add the potatoes, swede and parsnips, cover, then simmer for 10–15 more minutes or until the vegetables are tender. Drain and mash together, adding the milk, butter, salt and pepper. Spoon into a serving bowl and sprinkle the chives over. Garnish with the mint and serve.

Sweet and Sour Chicken with Brown Rice

Serves 2–3

Submitted by David Craggs-Hinton

75 g (3 oz) brown rice, cooked
175 g (6 oz) chicken breast,
* skinned and cut into thin*
* strips*
pinch sea salt or to taste
pinch freshly ground black
* pepper or to taste*
1 tsp olive oil
15 g (½ oz) root ginger, peeled
* and grated*
2–3 sprigs fresh coriander
¼ tsp Chinese five-spice powder
1 garlic clove, crushed
2 tsp demerara sugar
300 ml (½ pint) filtered water

50 g (2 oz) green beans, sliced
50 g (2 oz) carrots, cut into
* 5-cm (2-in) long sticks*
50 g (2 oz) white cabbage, cut
* into 5-cm (2-in) long strips*
50 g (2 oz) beanshoots, cut
* diagonally into 2.5-cm (1-in)*
* lengths*
25 g (1 oz) water chestnuts,
* sliced*
2 tsp cider vinegar
1 tbsp soy sauce
15 g (½ oz) fresh basil,
* chopped, or pinch dried*

Place the chicken strips in a wok or frying pan and season with salt and pepper. Add the olive oil, cover and sauté for 5 minutes. Add the ginger, coriander, Chinese five-spice powder, garlic, sugar and half of the water. Bring to the boil and simmer gently for 5 minutes. Remove the chicken and keep warm. Now add to the pan the green beans, carrots, cabbage, beanshoots, water chestnuts, cider vinegar and soy sauce to taste. Gradually pour in the remaining water, stirring well. Cover and cook until the vegetables are soft and the stock has reduced. Add the chicken once more and stir well. Serve on a ring of brown rice and garnish with the chopped basil.

Salmon with Spinach and Pasta

Serves 2–3

Submitted by David Craggs-Hinton

2 x 100-g (4-oz) salmon steaks
2 pinches sea salt or to taste
pinch freshly ground black
  pepper or to taste
15 g (½ oz) butter
550 ml (18 fl oz) skimmed milk
  or rice milk
2 sprigs fresh basil or pinch
  dried mixed herbs

175 g (6 oz) fresh spinach,
  finely chopped
2 tsp cornflour
175 g (6 oz) wholemeal pasta,
  cooked, drained and rinsed
25 g (1 oz) Parmesan cheese
  or to taste, finely grated
2 sprigs fresh parsley

Place the salmon in a medium saucepan, add a pinch of salt, pepper, the butter, half of the milk and the basil or mixed herbs, cover and poach for 15–20 minutes or until the salmon is cooked. Place the spinach in a medium saucepan with a pinch of salt, cover with water, bring to the boil, cover and simmer for 10 minutes. Remove the salmon from the milk and keep warm. Pour the remaining milk into the pan, add the cornflour and bring to the boil, stirring continuously, until the sauce thickens. Drain the spinach and add to the hot pasta. Add the sauce to the pasta and spinach and stir well. Garnish each serving with a sprinkling of Parmesan cheese and a sprig of parsley. Serve.

Tunisian Vegetable Couscous

Serves 6–8

275 g (10 oz) wholewheat
  couscous
400 ml (14 fl oz) boiling
  filtered water
1 large onion, finely chopped
2 garlic cloves, crushed
2 tbsp white wine
500-g (16-oz) tin tomatoes,
  chopped
3 large carrots, cut into 2.5-
  cm (1-in) long sticks
2 large celery sticks, cut into
  2.5-cm (1-in) long sticks
1 medium turnip, cut into 1-cm
  (½-in) dice
½ tsp ground cinnamon

½ tsp turmeric
1 tsp paprika
pinch cayenne pepper or to
  taste
2 tsp dark corn syrup
225 g (½ lb) aubergine, cut into
  2.5-cm (1-in) strips
1 red bell pepper, deseeded
  and chopped
75 g (3 oz) raisins
150 g (5 oz) dried apricots,
  chopped
300-g (11-oz) tin chickpeas,
  drained and rinsed
4 sprigs fresh mint or parsley,
  chopped

Place the couscous in a large bowl and add the boiling water. Let it stand for 15 minutes, then fluff with a fork and keep warm. Sauté the onion and garlic in the wine until limp. Add the tomatoes and their liquid, carrots, celery, turnip, spices and corn syrup and bring to the boil. Cover and simmer for about 20 minutes. Add the aubergine, red pepper, raisins, apricots and chickpeas. Cover and simmer for an additional 15 minutes. Place the couscous in individual soup bowls and top with the vegetable stew. Garnish with the chopped mint or parsley.

Pesto Sauce for Pasta

Serves 4–6

225 g (8 oz) wholemeal pasta,
    cooked and drained
2 large garlic cloves, raw or
    roasted
2 tbsp olive oil
1 large bunch fresh basil
    leaves

75 g (3 oz) shelled walnuts
1 tbsp soy sauce
8–14 tbsp filtered water, as
    required
pinch sea salt or to taste
pinch freshly ground black
    pepper or to taste

Place the garlic and olive oil in a blender or food processor and mix until the garlic has been pulverized. Add the remaining ingredients to the blender or food processor, keeping back a few sprigs of basil. Using 8 tablespoons of water, blend the mixture until smooth, adding more water as required. Pour over the hot wholemeal pasta, garnishing with the remaining basil. Serve.

Spaghetti Balls

Serves 4–6

600 g (20 oz) wholemeal
    spaghetti
350 g (12 oz) tofu, squeezed to
    remove liquid
1 small onion, finely chopped
50 g (2 oz) wholemeal
    breadcrumbs
1½ tbsp unsweetened peanut
    butter

2 tbsp soy sauce
1 garlic clove, crushed
½ tsp mustard powder
1 tbsp filtered water
pinch freshly ground black
    pepper or to taste
2 tsp olive oil
15 g (½ oz) fresh parsley, finely
    chopped

Bring a large pan of water to the boil, add the spaghetti, stirring, once the strands have softened, to separate them. Cook for about 10–15 minutes until tender, then drain. Meanwhile, place the tofu in a mixing bowl and mash with a fork. Using a wooden spoon, mix in all the other ingredients, except for the oil and a little of the parsley. Coat a heavy-bottomed frying pan with the olive oil and heat. Shape the mixture into small balls and brown on all sides over a medium heat. Drain on a paper towel and serve on the pasta. Garnish with the remaining parsley.

Fettucine with Lentil Sauce

Serves 4

450 g (1 lb) dried or fresh
  fettucine or tagliatelle
2 tbsp olive oil
2 garlic cloves, crushed
1 large onion, finely chopped
225 g (8 oz) red lentils,
  washed and drained

3 tbsp tomato purée
300 ml (½ pint) boiling filtered
  water
pinch sea salt or to taste
pinch freshly ground black
  pepper or to taste
4 sprigs fresh parsley, chopped

Place the pasta in a large saucepan, cover with water and cook according to the directions on the packaging. Drain, rinse and set aside. Heat the olive oil, then sauté the garlic and onion for 2 minutes, stirring occasionally. Add the lentils, tomato purée, salt and pepper, then stir in the boiling water. Bring to the boil, cover and simmer, stirring occasionally, for about 20 minutes or until the lentils are soft. Add more water if it looks too dry. Season with the salt and pepper. Reheat the pasta if necessary, then serve topped with the sauce. Garnish with the parsley.

Baked Macaroni with Béchamel Sauce

Serves 4

450 g (1 lb) wholemeal
  macaroni, cooked
3 tbsp sunflower or sesame oil
2 medium onions, chopped
1 large carrot, sliced into 2.5-
  cm (1-in) long sticks
3 tbsp organic wholemeal flour

450 ml (¾ pint) filtered water
225 g (½ lb) firm tofu, drained
  and crumbled
4 tbsp soy sauce or to taste
1 tbsp toasted sesame seeds
  (optional)
4 sprigs fresh thyme, chopped

Preheat the oven to 180°C (350°F, gas mark 4). Heat the oil in a large saucepan and sauté the onions and carrot for 5 minutes, until the onions have become transparent and lightly browned. Lower the heat and gradually stir in the flour. Brown lightly for 30 seconds, stirring constantly. Slowly pour in the water, stirring all the time to prevent lumps forming. Return to a medium heat and cook, stirring until smooth and thickened. Now stir in the tofu and season with soy sauce. Place the cooked macaroni in a large casserole dish and stir in the vegetables and sauce, making sure the macaroni is all coated with sauce. Top with sesame seeds, if using. Cover and cook in the preheated oven for 20 minutes. Remove the lid and cook for a further 20 minutes. Take out of the oven and allow to rest for 10 minutes before serving. Garnish with the chopped thyme.

Almond and Mushroom Casserole

Serves 4

225 g (½ lb) wholemeal pasta,
  cooked
5 tbsp sunflower oil
2 tbsp organic wholemeal flour
250 ml (8 fl oz) unsweetened
  soya milk
2 tbsp chopped fresh parsley
1 tsp fresh lemon juice
½ tsp celery salt
225 g (½ lb) firm tofu, squeezed
  to remove excess water

225 g (½ lb) mushrooms,
  chopped
½ large green bell pepper,
  deseeded and finely chopped
225 g (½ lb) blanched flaked
  almonds
100 g (4 oz) wholemeal
  breadcrumbs

Preheat the oven to 190°C (375°F, gas mark 5). Heat 3 tablespoons of the oil in a large saucepan over a medium heat. Add the flour, stirring until it absorbs the oil and is just starting to brown. Gradually pour in the milk, stirring or whisking constantly to avoid lumps forming. Continue cooking and stirring until the sauce begins to thicken. Remove from the heat and stir in the parsley, lemon juice and celery salt. Crumble in the tofu, mixing well, then set the sauce aside. Heat the remaining oil in a small frying pan, adding the mushrooms and sautéing until tender. Mix the mushrooms, green pepper, almonds and cooked pasta into the sauce. Transfer the mixture to a casserole dish, spreading evenly. Sprinkle the breadcrumbs over the pasta mixture and bake in the preheated oven for about 20 minutes. Remove when the top has lightly browned. Serve hot.

Pasta Oregano

Serves 2

Submitted by David Craggs-Hinton

350 g (12 oz) wholemeal
pasta, cooked and drained
1 small red onion, finely
chopped
2 tsp olive oil
750 g (1½ lbs) fresh plum
tomatoes, roughly chopped
1 red bell pepper, deseeded
and chopped
1 orange bell pepper, deseeded
and chopped
50 g (2 oz) green olives,
stoned and chopped

1–2 garlic cloves to taste
½ tsp dried oregano
2 tsp tomato purée
½ tbsp organic cider vinegar
pinch sea salt or to taste
pinch freshly ground black
pepper or to taste
15 g (½ oz) fresh thyme,
chopped
50 g (2 oz) Parmesan cheese,
finely grated

Place the onion in a frying pan with the olive oil and a little of the juice from the tomatoes. Sauté until the onions have become transparent. Add the peppers, olives and garlic and cook for a further 5 minutes. Add the oregano, tomatoes, tomato purée, cider vinegar, salt and pepper and bring to the boil. Simmer for 20–30 minutes. Top the pasta with the sauce, sprinkle with the thyme and Parmesan cheese and serve.

Pasta Primavera

Serves 4

350 g (12 oz) wholemeal
  spaghetti, cooked and
  drained
2 tbsp sunflower oil
1 bunch spring onions, thinly
  sliced, green and white parts
  in separate piles
225 g (8 oz) carrots, sliced
  into 2.5-cm (1-in) long sticks

2 medium aubergines, sliced
  into 2.5-cm (1-in) long sticks
225 g (8 oz) fresh or frozen
  garden peas
2 tbsp fresh mint leaves,
  chopped
pinch sea salt or to taste
pinch freshly ground black
  pepper or to taste

Heat the oil in a large saucepan over a medium heat. Add the white parts of the spring onions and sauté very gently for 2–3 minutes. Add the carrots and lower the heat. Cover and simmer for 5 minutes, then add the aubergines and peas, covering and simmering for a further 2–3 minutes. Turn off the heat, stir in the mint and season with salt and pepper. Transfer the cooked vegetables to the saucepan or dish in which you have the spaghetti and mix together. Serve hot.

Lazy Mini Pizzas

Serves 3–6

1 tbsp olive oil
1 red onion, chopped
1 tsp dried mixed herbs
1 tsp dried oregano
pinch garlic salt
3 tomatoes, skinned
6 green olives, stoned
*100 g (4 oz) tinned kidney
   beans, drained and roughly
   chopped*

*3 fresh soft wholemeal rolls,
   halved*
pinch sea salt or to taste
*pinch freshly ground black
   pepper or to taste*
*40 g (1½ oz) Edam cheese,
   grated*

Place the olive oil in a medium frying pan and add the onion. Sauté for 2 minutes, then add the herbs and garlic salt. Sauté for a further 2 minutes, then add the tomatoes, olives and beans. Cover and simmer for 10 minutes. Toast the outsides of the rolls, then spread the tomato mixture evenly on the cut surface of each half, seasoning with the salt and pepper. Place on a baking tray, sprinkle the cheese on top of the mixture and grill until the cheese has turned golden and is bubbling. Serve, with a side salad if desired.

No-fry Chips

Serves 1–2

1 large potato, peeled and chipped

Place the chips on a microwave-safe plate in a radial fashion, with the end of each chip pointing towards the centre of the plate. Microwave on high for 2 minutes, flipping them over and removing any that are cooked. Microwave for a further 2 minutes or until the chips are pliable but not too dried. Place on a lightly oiled baking tray and grill for a few minutes, turning them over so that all sides become browned. Serve hot.

Sweet Potato Chips

Serves 3

2 sweet potatoes (or yams), peeled and chipped
olive oil as required
½ tsp garlic salt

Preheat the oven to 180°C (350°F, gas mark 4). Place the chips on a lightly oiled baking tray and brush on a light coating of olive oil. Sprinkle with some of the garlic salt and bake for 20 minutes in the preheated oven. Turn the chips over, sprinkle with the remaining garlic salt and bake for another 10 minutes. Serve hot.

Cajun Fish Fillets

Serves 4

450 g (1 lb) any white fish
1 tsp cajun spice
1 tbsp paprika
pinch freshly ground black
    pepper or to taste

1 lemon, quartered
salad, Sweet Potato Chips or
    No-fry Chips (page 108) to
    serve

Arrange the fillets on a lightly oiled grill pan. Mix together the cajun spice and paprika and sprinkle over the fillets so they are well coated. Grill close to the heat for 5–6 minutes or until the spices have browned and the fish is firm and will flake with a fork. Season with black pepper and serve with a salad, Sweet Potato Chips or No-fry Chips (page 108). Garnish with the lemon wedges.

Kedgeree

Serves 4

225 g (8 oz) haddock, smoked
    or unsmoked
1 small onion, finely chopped
1 dsp olive oil

175 g (6 oz) organic long-
    grain brown rice
pinch cayenne pepper
4 sprigs fresh parsley, chopped

Place the haddock in a medium saucepan and cover with water. Poach gently for 10 minutes, then drain, reserving the liquid. Remove the bones and skin from the fish, flaking the flesh loosely with a fork. Sauté the onion in the oil until soft, add the rice and cayenne pepper, then stir for a few more seconds. Mix in the liquid from the fish and simmer until the rice is tender (about 30 minutes), adding more water if required. Stir frequently. Gently add the flaked haddock and mix together. Turn on to a heated dish, garnish with the parsley and serve.

Caribbean Pork and Pineapple

Serves 2–3

*175 g (6 oz) brown rice,
  cooked*
*275 g (10 oz) pork tenderloin,
  chopped into large dice*
*100 g (4 oz) onion, finely
  chopped*
100 g (4 oz) mushrooms, sliced
*100 g (4 oz) pineapple cubes
  in natural juice*

*150 ml (¼-pint) vegetable stock
  or Home-made Vegetable
  Stock (page 85)*
150 ml (¼-pint) tomato juice
*15 g (½ oz) fresh ginger root,
  peeled and finely chopped
  (optional)*
2 sprigs fresh basil

Place the pork and onions in a frying pan and sauté gently until the pork has sealed on all sides and the onions have softened, adding a teaspoonful of water if the onion begins to stick. Add the remaining ingredients, except the basil, cover and simmer for 20–25 minutes. Serve on a ring of brown rice and garnish with the basil.

Beef Casserole

Serves 4

*450 g (1 lb) lean braising
  steak, cut into strips*
350 g (½ oz) carrots, sliced
225 g (8 oz) leeks, sliced
350 g (12 oz) swede
100 g (4 oz) pearl barley

*900 ml (1½ pints) vegetable
  stock or Home-made
  Vegetable Stock (page 85)*
pinch sea salt or to taste
*jacket potato and green beans
  to serve*

Preheat the oven to 170°C (325°F, gas mark 3). Place all the ingredients in a saucepan, cover with water and bring to the boil. Skim the excess fat from the top, then stir and place in a casserole dish. Cover and cook in the preheated oven for 1½–2 hours. Serve with the jacket potato and green beans.

Chicken Burgers

Serves 4

225 g (8 oz) cooked chicken
   breast, minced
1 small onion, grated
small pinch sea salt
pinch freshly ground black
   pepper or to taste

275 g (10 oz) cottage cheese,
   sieved to remove the liquid
1 tsp mixed herbs
salad to serve

Place the chicken and the onion in a medium mixing bowl and mix together. Season with salt and pepper. Stir in the cottage cheese and mixed herbs, then make into 4 burger shapes. Leave to cool in a refrigerator for 1–2 hours before cooking under a hot grill for about 5 minutes each side or until the burgers are a golden colour. Serve with a salad.

Aubergine with Chicken Strips

Serves 4

1 tsp coriander seeds, roasted and finely ground	*350-g (12-oz) chicken fillet, cut into thin strips*
1 tsp fennel seeds, roasted and finely ground	*3 x 13-cm (5-in) long aubergines, sliced in half and cut into strips lengthways*
1 garlic clove, crushed	
1 tsp grated fresh ginger root	
pinch sea salt or to taste	*½ tsp tamari*
pinch freshly ground black pepper or to taste	*2 tsp brown rice vinegar*
2 tbsp olive oil, plus extra for aubergines	*salad or steamed vegetables to serve*

Preheat the oven to 200°C (400°F, gas mark 6). Combine the coriander and fennel seeds, garlic, ginger, salt and pepper with the olive oil in a blender or food processor. Mix until smooth. Half fill a large saucepan with water and bring to the boil. Blanch the chicken strips for 20 seconds, then immediately drain in a colander and plunge into a large bowl of ice-cold water. Leave in the cold water for about 10 minutes or until the strips have completely cooled. Drain again. Stir the chicken into the spicy oil mixture, then place in the refrigerator to marinate for at least 30 minutes. Slice each piece of aubergine across diagonally and rub with a little olive oil. Arrange them in a single layer in a large, lightly oiled ovenproof dish. Fill the gaps with the marinated chicken strips. Cook in the preheated oven for 7–8 minutes. Turn the oven off without opening the door and leave the dish to stand for a further 3–4 minutes. Ensure the chicken strips are cooked through. Sprinkle with the tamari and rice vinegar, then serve while still hot with a salad or steamed vegetables.

Spinach and Lentil Stew

Serves 5

1 onion, chopped
50 ml (2 fl oz) vegetable stock
  or Home-made Vegetable
  Stock (page 85)
4 garlic cloves, finely chopped
175 g (6 oz) split red lentils,
  rinsed
400-g (14-oz) tin chopped
  tomatoes, with juice
4 tsp stock granules
1 tbsp Worcestershire sauce

1 tsp dried thyme
½ tsp ground fennel seeds
  (optional)
1 bay leaf
pinch sea salt or to taste
2 medium carrots, diced
275 g (10 oz) fresh or frozen spinach,
  chopped
900 ml (1½ pints) filtered water
1 tbsp organic apple cider
  vinegar

Place the onion in a large saucepan and sauté in the vegetable stock until soft (3–4 minutes). Add the garlic, lentils, tomatoes and juice, stock granules, Worcestershire sauce, thyme, fennel seeds, if using, bay leaf and salt, together with the water. Bring to the boil, cover and, stirring occasionally, simmer for 20 minutes or until the lentils start to break up. Add the carrots and spinach and stir well (if the spinach was frozen, stir until it has thawed). Cover and simmer for a further 15 minutes or until the carrots and spinach are cooked. Remove the bay leaf and stir in the vinegar. Serve hot.

Potato Gnocchi

Serves 4

3 large baking potatoes,
  pricked
150 g (5 oz) organic
  wholemeal self-raising flour

½ tsp sea salt
1 x Tangy Pasta Sauce recipe
  (below) to serve

Bake or microwave the potatoes until tender, allowing them to rest at room temperature until they are cool enough to handle. Scoop the potato out of the skins and mash in a bowl. Add the flour and salt, mixing in well, then turn the mixture on to a floured surface. Knead until smooth, adding more flour if necessary so the 'dough' does not stick. Bring a large saucepan of water to the boil. Form the dough into 2-cm (¾-in) thick sausages, then cut across at 2-cm (¾-in) intervals. Press the top of each shape lightly with a fork to create stripes. Add the gnocchi to the boiling water, boiling until they float to the top. Remove them from the water and drain well. Place in a large bowl, adding sufficient Tangy Pasta Sauce to lightly coat all the gnocchi. Serve with additional Tangy Pasta Sauce.

Tangy Pasta Sauce

Serves 4

1 tbsp olive oil
1 onion, finely chopped
1 large garlic clove, crushed
1 bell pepper, any colour,
  deseeded and finely chopped
1 small aubergine, sliced,
  slices cut in half
1 kg (2¼ lbs) fresh plum
  tomatoes, coarsely chopped

1 tbsp fresh basil, chopped
pinch sea salt or to taste
pinch freshly ground black
  pepper or to taste
2 tsp fresh coriander, chopped
1 x Potato Gnocchi recipe
  (above) to serve

Heat the oil in a large, heavy bottomed saucepan over a medium heat. Add the onion and garlic, then sauté for 5 minutes. Add the bell pepper and aubergine and continue to sauté until the onions have become tender. Add the tomatoes, basil, salt and pepper and simmer gently for a further 25 minutes. Garnish with the chopped coriander and serve with Potato Gnocchi.

Vegetable Paella

Serves 1

50 g (2 oz) brown rice
250 ml (8 fl oz) boiling filtered
water
1 small onion, chopped
1 small green bell pepper,
deseeded and chopped
2 small tomatoes, roughly
chopped
25 g (1 oz) mushrooms, chopped

3 tbsp sweetcorn, drained if
tinned
½ tsp dried thyme or marjoram
1 tsp lemon juice or to taste
1 tsp soy sauce or to taste
pinch freshly ground black
pepper or to taste
25 g (1 oz) peanuts, crushed,
or peanut butter (optional)

Place the rice in a medium saucepan with the boiling water. Bring back to the boil, cover and leave to simmer for 10 minutes. Add the vegetables, except the sweetcorn, to the rice, stir, cover and simmer for 15 minutes. Stir in the sweetcorn, herbs, lemon juice and soy sauce. Season with the pepper, cover and simmer for a further 5 minutes. If using peanut butter, stir it in at this point. If using peanuts, sprinkle them on top of the dish. Serve hot.

Modern Ratatouille

Serves 4–6

1 onion, chopped
1 green bell pepper, deseeded
and chopped
4 garlic cloves, crushed
6 large tomatoes, peeled and
deseeded
2 tsp mixed spice

85 ml (3 fl oz) vegetable stock
or Home-made Vegetable
Stock (page 85), plus extra
as required
4 medium aubergines, sliced
15 g (½ oz) fresh basil,
chopped, or pinch dried
juice of 1 lemon

Place the onion, pepper and garlic in a wok or large frying pan and sauté for 5 minutes or until soft. Add the tomatoes, mixed spice and stock. Cover and simmer for 20 minutes, stirring occasionally and adding more stock if necessary. Add the aubergines, basil and lemon juice and simmer for another 5–10 minutes, until the aubergine has become tender but is still bright. Serve.

Rice Pilaf

Serves 2

175 ml (6 fl oz) vegetable or chicken stock
175 g (6 oz) long-grain brown rice
25 g (1 oz) diced celery

25 g (1 oz) deseeded and diced green bell pepper
1 small onion, finely chopped
2 tbsp fresh parsley, chopped

Place the stock, rice, celery, pepper and onion in a large saucepan and bring to the boil. Cover and simmer for 20 minutes or until all the liquid has been absorbed and the rice is tender. Stir in the parsley just before serving.

Chicken Rolls

Serves 2

Submitted by Margaret Gray

1 slice wholemeal bread
1 tbsp filtered water
1 small onion, finely chopped
1 dsp fresh sage or pinch dried
pinch sea salt or to taste

pinch freshly ground black pepper or to taste
1 small organic free-range egg
2 chicken fillets, skinned, washed and patted dry
steamed vegetables to serve

Preheat the oven to 240°C (475°F, gas mark 9). Place the bread in a bowl and rub until small crumbs are formed. Add the water and set aside. Microwave the onion on high for 2 minutes or until it has softened, then drain. Make a hollow in the breadcrumb mixture and add the onion, sage, salt and pepper and mix well. Add the egg and mix again. Place the chicken pieces in a lightly oiled oven-proof dish and spread the bread mixture generously on top. Roll the chicken, ensuring that the 'stuffing' stays in the middle, and secure with cocktail sticks or string. Bake in the preheated oven for about 15 minutes or until the chicken is tender. Serve with steamed vegetables.

Avocado and Cheese

Serves 2

Submitted by Margaret Gray

2 ripe avocados
100 g (4 oz) cottage cheese
1 tbsp fat-free mayonnaise
185-g (7-oz) tin salmon or
    tuna
½ small onion, finely chopped

½ tsp freshly squeezed lemon
    juice
pinch paprika
1 hard-boiled free-range egg,
    sliced
mixed green salad and
    wholemeal rolls to serve

Cut the avocados in half lengthways, remove the stone and spoon out the flesh into a bowl, leaving just the skins – set these to one side. Add the cottage cheese, mayonnaise, fish, onion and lemon juice to the bowl with the avocado and mix together with either a fork or blender until smooth. Spoon the mixture into the skins. Sprinkle with the paprika and garnish with the egg slices. Serve with a mixed green salad and wholemeal rolls.

Avocado Vinaigrette

Serves 4

4 tsp organic apple cider
    vinegar
6 tbsp olive oil
pinch sea salt or to taste

pinch freshly ground black
    pepper or to taste
2 ripe avocados
salad to serve, if not a starter

Place the vinegar, olive oil and seasonings in a bowl and mix together. Chill in the refrigerator until ready to serve. Cut the avocados in half lengthways and remove the stones. Place on plates and fill the hollows with the vinaigrette. Serve as a starter or with a salad.

Pasta 'n' Fish

Serves 2

Submitted by Margaret Gray

*225 g (8 oz) fresh haddock or
   cod
soya or rice milk as required
100 g (4 oz) wholemeal pasta
100 g (4 oz) low-fat organic
   cheese, grated*

*1 x Home-made Coleslaw
   recipe (below) and salad to
   serve*

Preheat the oven to 230°C (450°F, gas mark 8). Poach the fish in a little soya or rice milk, enough to cover. Remove any skin and bones, flake and set to one side. Add the pasta to a pan of boiling water and simmer for 12 minutes. Place the fish and pasta in an ovenproof dish and mix together. Stir in the cheese, saving some for later. Place in the preheated oven and bake for 5–10 minutes or until the cheese has melted and the top browned. Sprinkle the remaining cheese over the top and serve with the Home-made Coleslaw and salad.

Home-made Coleslaw

Serves 4–8

Submitted by Margaret Gray

*½ small white cabbage, finely
   chopped
1 small carrot, finely chopped
1 celery stick, finely chopped*

*25 g (1 oz) raisins or nuts
175–225 g (6–8 oz) fat-free
   mayonnaise*

Place the dry ingredients in a bowl and mix well. Add the mayonnaise and stir again. Good served with the Pasta 'n' Fish (above) or a salad or baked potato.

Stuffed Eggs

Serves 2–4

Submitted by Margaret Gray

4 eggs, soft-boiled and shelled
1 x 185-g (7-oz) tin sardines
*   or tuna*
1 tbsp fat-free mayonnaise
pinch sea salt or to taste

pinch freshly ground black
*   pepper or to taste*
25 g (1 oz) watercress
salad and wholemeal bread to
*   serve*

Cut the eggs lengthways and spoon the yolks into a bowl. Add the sardines or tuna, mayonnaise and salt and pepper. Mix well, then spoon the mixture into the hollows in the egg whites, piling it up. Garnish with the watercress. Serve with a salad and wholemeal bread.

Nut Pâté

Serves 3–4

Submitted by Margaret Gray

50 g (2 oz) almonds
50 g (2 oz) sunflower seeds
50 g (2 oz) cashew nuts,
*   broken*
120–175 ml (4–6 fl oz)
*   vegetable stock or Home-*
*   made Vegetable Stock*
*   (page 85)*

salad or jacket potatoes or
*   wholemeal bread or crackers*
*   to serve*

Place all the ingredients in a blender or food processor and grind to a powder. Add sufficient stock to make a paste. Turn into a freezer-proof plastic container and freeze for 2 or more hours before serving. Serve with the salad, jacket potatoes, bread or crackers.

Bean Pâté

Serves 3

*350-g (12-oz) tin red kidney
   beans*
1 garlic clove, crushed
1 tbsp tomato purée
1 tsp organic soy sauce
1 tsp fresh lemon juice

½ tsp Tabasco sauce
pinch sea salt or to taste
*pinch freshly ground black
   pepper or to taste*
salad or baked potato to serve

Drain the kidney beans, reserving the liquid. Place all the beans and
the rest of the ingredients in a large bowl and mash with a fork.
Beat well with a wooden spoon or use a food processor. If necessary,
add a little of the liquid from the beans to make the mixture into a
thick paste. Adjust the seasoning to taste, then spoon into medium
ramekins and chill in the refrigerator for about 30 minutes before
serving. Serve with the salad or baked potato.

Salads

Bulgar Wheat Salad with Herbs and Walnuts

Serves 4

225 g (8 oz) bulgar wheat
350 ml (½ fl oz) vegetable
stock or Home-made
Vegetable Stock (page 85)
pinch ground cumin
1 cinnamon stick
pinch cayenne pepper
pinch ground cloves
1 red bell pepper, roasted,
skinned, deseeded and diced
1 yellow bell pepper, roasted,
skinned, deseeded and diced
2 plum tomatoes, roasted,
skinned, deseeded and diced

2 shallots, finely chopped
25 g (1 oz) mangetout, topped
and tailed
5 black olives, stoned and
quartered
50 g (2 oz) walnuts, roughly
chopped
2 tbsp chopped fresh basil,
parsley and mint
2 tbsp lemon juice
2 tbsp olive oil
pinch freshly ground black
pepper or to taste

Place the bulgar wheat in a large bowl. Pour the stock into a saucepan, adding the cumin, cinnamon, cayenne pepper and ground cloves. Bring to the boil and simmer for 1 minute. Pour over the bulgar wheat and allow to stand for 30 minutes. Meanwhile, place the peppers, tomatoes, shallots, mangetout, olives, walnuts and herbs in another bowl and add the lemon juice, olive oil and black pepper. Stir well. Drain the bulgar wheat, shaking the sieve or colander well to remove excess water. Remove the cinnamon stick and pour the bulgar wheat into a large serving bowl. Stir in the fresh vegetable mixture and serve.

Black Bean Salad

Serves 6

175 g (6 oz) organic long-
   grain brown rice
175 ml (6 fl oz) vegetable
   stock or Home-made
   Vegetable Stock (page 85)
175 g (6 oz) pineapple chunks,
   chopped
450-g (15-oz) tin black beans,
   drained and rinsed
1 red bell pepper, deseeded
   and diced
2 celery sticks, diced

1 medium onion, finely
   chopped
3 tbsp organic cider vinegar
2 tbsp olive oil
2 tsp Dijon mustard
1 tsp muscovado or demerara
   sugar or to taste
pinch sea salt or to taste
pinch freshly ground black
   pepper or to taste

Place the rice and stock in a medium saucepan and bring to the boil. Stir, cover and simmer for 30 minutes. Keep covered, but remove the pan from the heat and allow to stand for 5 minutes, then fluff with a fork. Add the pineapple, beans, pepper, celery and onion and toss to combine. Add the remaining ingredients and toss to coat the salad. Serve.

Tangy Sweet Potato Salad with Chickpeas

Serves 6

4 sweet potatoes, peeled and
  cut into 2.5-cm (1-in) cubes
100 g (4 oz) cooked or tinned
  chickpeas, drained
1 tbsp red onion, finely
  chopped
1 tbsp olive oil
25 g (1 oz) organic cider
  vinegar

1 tbsp Dijon mustard
2 tsp raw honey
2 tsp Worcestershire sauce
pinch sea salt or to taste
pinch freshly ground black
  pepper or to taste

Place the sweet potatoes in a large saucepan and cover with water. Bring to the boil, cover and simmer for 10 minutes or until just tender. Drain and set aside to cool to room temperature. Combine the cooled potatoes with the chickpeas and onion in a medium bowl. Place the remaining ingredients in a small bowl and whisk together. Spoon the dressing over the potato mixture and toss gently to coat all the ingredients.

Artichoke Salad

Serves 6

400-g (14-oz) tin artichoke
  hearts, drained and sliced
3 large tomatoes, sliced
1 green bell pepper, deseeded
  and diced
15 g (½ oz) fresh parsley, finely
  chopped, or pinch dried

6 tbsp olive oil
2 tbsp organic cider vinegar
1 garlic clove, crushed
pinch sea salt or to taste
pinch freshly ground black
  pepper or to taste

Place the artichoke hearts in a salad bowl with the tomatoes and pepper. Season to taste. Mix the remaining ingredients together in another small bowl. Pour over the salad and chill for 10 minutes before serving.

Desserts

Lemon Mousse

Serves 8

550 ml (18 fl oz) pineapple
juice
85 ml (3 fl oz) orange juice
concentrate
75 g (3 oz) arrowroot
1 tbsp lemon zest

6 tbsp lemon juice
6 tbsp honey or to taste
1 tbsp orange peel, cut into
thin strips
¼ tsp sea salt

Combine all the ingredients in a blender or food processor and mix until smooth. Pour the mixture into a saucepan and bring to the boil. Cover and simmer for 6–7 minutes, until thick, stirring all the time. Place in dessert glasses and chill in the refrigerator until cold and set. Serve.

Fruity Rice Pudding

Serves 3–4

175 ml (6 fl oz) rice milk
175 g (6 oz) brown rice,
cooked
75 g (3 oz) raisins
75 g (3 oz) dried apricots,
chopped

¼ tsp ground cinnamon
pinch ground cloves
pinch ground cardamom
(optional)

Place the rice milk in a medium saucepan and warm over a low heat. Stir in the remaining ingredients, cover and cook, without boiling, for 15–20 minutes, stirring occasionally. Remove when the fruits have become plump and soft and most of the milk has been absorbed. Serve hot.

Grapefruit Cups

Serves 4

2 grapefruit   ½ tsp fructose or fruit juice
2 glacé cherries, cut in half   sweetener

Cut the grapefruit in half, then cut around each half, loosening
the flesh from the outer skin. Cut between the segments to loosen
the flesh, then remove the central core and pips. Place a grapefruit
half in each of four individual sundae glasses. Sprinkle with a little
fructose or sweetener and place half a glacé cherry in the middle of
each grapefruit. Serve either as a starter or dessert.

Banana Split

Serves 2

2 bananas   100 g (4 oz) strawberries,
4 tsp low-fat fromage frais   hulled
4 tsp strawberry or banana
  tofu yogurt

Remove the skins from the bananas and cut each banana in half
lengthways. Mix together the yogurt and fromage frais and pile
half in the centre of each of two dessert plates. Place banana halves
along each side of the mixture for both plates. Liquidize the strawberries in a blender or food processor. Pour the resulting sauce over
the banana halves.

Fresh Fruit Salad

Serves 4

50 g (2 oz) cherries, stoned
50 g (2 oz) seedless grapes,
washed
1 red apple, unpeeled, washed,
cored and diced
1 green apple, unpeeled,
washed, cored and diced

1 orange, peeled and
segmented
2 apricots, diced
1 kiwi fruit, diced
juice of 1 lemon
150 ml (5 fl oz) unsweetened
apple juice

Place the cherries, grapes, apples, orange, apricots and kiwi fruit in a bowl and mix together. Pour the lemon and apple juices over the fruit and refrigerate for at least 1 hour before serving.

Baked Apple with Sultanas

Serves 1

1 medium cooking apple,
washed, cored and lightly
punctured

pinch ground cinnamon
15 g (½ oz) sultanas

Preheat the oven to 200°C (400°F, gas mark 6). Fill the centre of the apple with sultanas and sprinkle the cinnamon over. Place the apple in an ovenproof dish and pour a little water around it. Bake in the preheated oven for 30–40 minutes. Allow to cool for a few minutes before serving.

Cakes and biscuits

Farmhouse Biscuits

Makes about 20 biscuits

175 g (6 oz) organic
  wholemeal self-raising flour
50 g (2 oz) fine oatmeal
100 g (4 oz) butter
25 g (1 oz) demerara sugar

1 tsp baking powder
½ tsp celery salt
½ tsp cayenne pepper
1 tbsp skimmed milk

Preheat the oven to 180°C (350°F, gas mark 4). Place all the dry ingredients in a bowl and mix, rubbing in the butter. Add the milk slowly, mixing until a soft dough forms. Roll out the dough on a floured surface until it is 3 mm (⅛-in) thick. Using a biscuit cutter, cut out shapes and place them on a lightly oiled baking tray. Bake in the preheated oven for 15–20 minutes, until firm and golden. Cool on a wire rack, then store in an airtight container. (Due to the high butter content, try to make these biscuits a treat!)

Oatie Cake

Makes 1 cake

425 g (15 oz) fine oatmeal
75 g (3 oz) raisins
2 tbsp muscovado sugar
2 tsp baking powder
½ tsp ground cinnamon

175 ml (6 fl oz) rice milk
2 organic free-range eggs
pinch sea salt or to taste
75 g (3 oz) apple sauce
1 tsp vanilla essence

Preheat the oven to 180°C (350°F, gas mark 4). Place the dry ingredients in a bowl and mix. Place the wet ingredients in another bowl, whisk together, then stir into the dry ingredients. Turn the mixture into a lightly oiled 23-cm (9-in) cake tin and bake in the preheated oven for 20–30 minutes, until a skewer inserted in the centre comes out clean. Turn on to a wire rack and allow to cool before serving.

Mixed Fruit Teabread

Makes 1 loaf

175 g (6 oz) raisins
100 g (4 oz) sultanas
50 g (2 oz) currants
150 g (5 oz) muscovado or
  demerara sugar
300 ml (½ pint) strong cold
  black tea, strained

1 tbsp soya flour mixed with
  1 tbsp filtered water
225 g (8 oz) plain organic
  wholemeal flour
1½ tsp baking powder
½ tsp ground mixed spice

Preheat the oven to 180°C (350°F, gas mark 4). Place the dried fruit and sugar in a bowl and pour in the tea. Mix well, then soak overnight (or for at least 7 hours). The next day, add the soya flour and water mixture, flour, baking powder and mixed spice to the fruit and tea mixture. Mix thoroughly with a wooden spoon until all the ingredients are evenly combined. Spoon into a lightly oiled 900-g (2-lb) loaf tin lined with greaseproof paper and bake in the preheated oven for 1¼ hours or until the teabread has risen and a skewer inserted in the centre comes out almost clean. Turn the teabread out of the tin and allow it to cool on a wire rack. Wrap it in greaseproof paper and store in an airtight container for 1–2 days before eating.

Lemon Walnut Teabread

Makes 1 loaf or 24 muffins

75 g (3 oz) walnuts
350 g (12 oz) organic
   wholemeal self-raising flour
2 tsp baking powder
40 ml (1½ fl oz) fresh lemon
   juice
grated zest of 2 lemons

85 ml (3 fl oz) unsweetened
   apple juice
85 ml (3 fl oz) sunflower oil
85 ml (3 fl oz) golden syrup or
   maple syrup
pinch sea salt or to taste

Preheat the oven to 190°C (375°F, gas mark 5). Place the walnuts in a heavy bottomed frying pan and toast over a low heat for 5 minutes, stirring frequently. Remove and allow to cool, then chop. Place the lemon juice, lemon zest, apple juice, sunflower oil and golden or maple syrup in a large mixing bowl and beat together. In a separate bowl, mix the flour, baking powder and salt. Now mix the dry ingredients into the wet ingredients, stirring until the batter has become completely smooth. Fold in the walnuts. Pour the batter into a lightly oiled 900-g (2-lb) loaf tin or partially fill individual paper muffin or fairy cake cases in a muffin or fairy cake tray. Bake in the preheated oven for 15 minutes, then reduce the heat to 180°C (350°F, gas mark 4) and bake for an additional 20 minutes for a teabread, 15 minutes for muffins. Allow to cool before removing the teabread from the tin or the muffins from the tray. Serve warm or at room temperature.

Carrot Cake

Makes 1 large or 2 small cakes

550 g (1¼ lbs) brown rice flour (available from most healthfood shops)
4 tbsp tapioca, finely ground
1 tbsp linseeds, ground (available from healthfood shops)
225 g (8 oz) golden syrup or maple syrup
275 ml (9 fl oz) filtered water

350 g (12 oz) carrots, grated
175 g (6 oz) dried figs, finely chopped
1 baking apple, cooked and mashed
1 tbsp baking powder
3 tbsp prune purée
1 tbsp vanilla extract
pinch sea salt or to taste

Preheat the oven to 180°C (350°F, gas mark 4). Sift the flour, tapioca and linseeds together into a large mixing bowl. Combine the liquids, then stir into the flour mixture. Fold in the remaining ingredients, then pour into a lightly oiled cake tin 23 by 33 cm (9 by 13 in) or divide between two 25-cm (10-in) round tins. Bake in the preheated oven for 30–40 minutes (longer if using one tin). Turn on to a wire rack and allow to cool before serving.

Fig Bars

Makes about 9 bars

350 g (12 oz) dried figs,
  coarsely chopped
2 tsp freshly grated lemon zest
275 ml (9 fl oz) unsweetened
  apple juice
85 ml (3 fl oz) sunflower oil
50 g (2 oz) fructose or fruit
  juice sweetener

175 g (6 oz) self-raising
  organic wholemeal flour
175 g (6 oz) rolled oats (not
  instant oatmeal)
1 tsp baking powder
pinch sea salt or to taste

Preheat the oven to 180°C (350°F, gas mark 4). Place the figs, lemon zest and apple juice in a saucepan and bring to the boil. Lower the heat, cover and simmer gently for about 15 minutes, until the figs are tender. Remove from the heat and mash until smooth. Set aside. Place the sunflower oil and fructose or sweetener in a large bowl and mix together. Stir in the remaining ingredients, mixing to a crumb consistency. Press half the crumbly mixture into the bottom of a greaseproof paper-lined cake tin, topping with the fig mixture. Press the remaining crumbly mixture over the filling. Bake in the preheated oven for 40 minutes or until lightly browned. Allow to cool completely before cutting into bars.

Oatie Bran Fingers

Makes 18 fingers

225 g (8 oz) organic
  wholemeal flour
75 g (3 oz) rolled oats
75 g (3 oz) bran
150 g (5 oz) muscovado sugar

1 tsp ground ginger
1 tsp ground mixed spice
90 g (3½ oz) butter
275 ml (9 fl oz) skimmed milk

Preheat the oven to 180°C (350°F, gas mark 4). Place the flour, oats, bran, sugar and spices in a large bowl and mix. Add the butter and rub into the dry ingredients. Stir in the milk to make a stiff dough. Spoon into a greased 15 by 28-cm (6 by 11-in) cake tin and smooth the surface. Bake in the preheated oven for 25 minutes. Cool in the tin, then cut into bars to serve. Store in an airtight container and, due to their high butter content, try not to eat these too often!

Snacks

French Toast

Serves 4

1 baking apple, peeled and
   sliced
2 tbsp demerara sugar
3 tbsp linseeds (available
   from healthfood shops)

8 slices wholemeal bread
85 ml (3 fl oz) filtered water
175 ml (6 fl oz) unsweetened
   soya milk

Place the apple slices and sugar in a saucepan and add a little water. Bring to the boil, then simmer gently until the apple is tender. Drain, mash to make apple sauce and set to one side. Grind the linseeds in a blender until they turn to powder. Add the water and blend for 1 minute. Beat the linseed mixture into the soya milk. Dip the slices of bread in this mixture and cook until browned in a non-stick frying pan. Serve with the apple sauce.

Date Delight

Makes a plateful to share

Submitted by Margaret Gray

225 g (8 oz) dates, stoned
100 g (4 oz) cottage cheese

Widen the cavity in each date and fill with cottage cheese. Serve as a buffet snack or as a nibble to enjoy while watching TV.

Celery and Cheese

Makes a plateful to share

Submitted by Margaret Gray

4 celery sticks, washed and chopped into 5-cm (2-in) lengths
75 g (3 oz) cottage cheese
paprika, as required

Fill the grooves in the celery lengths with cottage cheese and sprinkle paprika over to taste. Serve as a buffet snack or as a TV nibble.

Fruit and Nut Mix

Makes 375 g (13 oz)

25 g (1 oz) dates, chopped
50 g (2 oz) raisins, washed
50 g (2 oz) unsalted cashews
50 g (2 oz) shelled pecans

50 g (2 oz) unsalted peanuts
50 g (2 oz) sunflower seeds
50 g (2 oz) hazelnuts (filberts)

Mix all the ingredients together and use for snacks. Keep in an airtight container. If stored in the freezer, it will keep for up to 3 months.

Breads

Wheatgerm Bread

Makes 2 loaves

4 tsp dried yeast
1 tsp caster sugar
600 ml (1 pint) warm filtered
    water
25 g (1 oz) butter
650 g (1 lb 6 oz) organic
    wholemeal flour

175 g (6 oz) wheatgerm
1 tsp sea salt
2 tsp malt extract
1 organic free-range egg,
    beaten

Blend the yeast with the sugar and a little of the warm water and leave for about 20 minutes until frothy. Rub the butter into the flour, wheatgerm, salt and malt extract, then make a well in the centre. Pour the yeast mixture into it, then stir it in, together with the remaining water, and mix to form a soft dough. Knead well until it is elastic and no longer sticky. Place the dough in an oiled bowl, cover with oiled clingfilm and leave in a warm place for about an hour, until it has doubled in size. Towards the end of this time, preheat the oven to 230°C (450°F, gas mark 8). Knead the dough again and divide between two greased 450-g (1-lb) loaf tins. Leave to rise in a warm place for about 40 minutes, until the dough rises just above the tops of the tins. Brush the tops of the loaves generously with the beaten egg. Bake in the preheated oven for about 30 minutes, until they are golden brown on top and sound hollow when tapped on the base.

Wholemeal Bread

Makes 1 loaf

150 g (5 oz) organic
  wholemeal flour
1 tbsp compressed yeast,
  loosely crumbled
1 tsp caster sugar
50 ml (2 fl oz) lukewarm
  filtered water

1 tsp sea salt
1 tsp honey
175 ml (6 fl oz) skimmed milk
sesame or poppy seeds to
  decorate

Place the yeast, sugar and lukewarm water in a bowl and mix. Stand in a warm place for 5–10 minutes until frothy. Mix the flour, salt and honey together in another bowl. Heat the milk gently until it is almost blood temperature, then add the yeast and the milk to flour mixture and stir thoroughly with a wooden spoon until mixed. Knead on a lightly floured surface for 10 minutes or until the dough becomes firm and pliable. Place it in an oiled bowl, covered with oiled clingfilm, and stand in a warm place for 40 minutes or until the dough has doubled in size. Set the oven to 220°C (425°F, gas mark 7), then knead the dough lightly, mould into the desired shape and stand in a warm place for 10–15 minutes. Sprinkle with sesame or poppy seeds. Bake in the oven for 30 minutes.

Banana Bread

Makes 1 cake

5 very ripe to overripe
  bananas
2 tbsp muscovado sugar
1 tsp vanilla extract
350 g (12 oz) organic
  wholemeal flour

2 tsp baking powder
½ tsp bicarbonate of soda
50 g (2 oz) dried fruit
  (optional)

Preheat the oven to 180°C (350°F, gas mark 4). Place the bananas, sugar and vanilla in a bowl or blender and mix until smooth. Place the remaining ingredients in another bowl and mix. Add the banana mixture to the dry ingredients and stir well. Spoon into a lightly oiled 20–25-cm (8–10-in) cake tin and bake in the preheated oven for about 1 hour or until a skewer inserted in the centre comes out almost clean. Turn on to a wire rack and allow to cool.

Drinks

Fruit Shake

Serves 2–3

1 apple, peeled, cored and
    chopped
75 g (3 oz) cherries, stoned
75 g (3 oz) peaches, peeled,
    stoned and sliced

1 small carton natural live
    yogurt
50 ml (2 fl oz) pineapple,
    apple or orange juice

Place all the ingredients in a blender, reserving 2 or 3 peach slices or cherries and mix until smooth. Pour into glasses and top with the peach slices or cherries.

Tangy Pink

Serves 2–3

1 pink grapefruit, peeled and segmented
1 blood orange, peeled and segmented
2 tbsp fresh lemon juice

Place the grapefruit and orange segments in a blender and mix. Stir in the lemon juice and pour into glasses.

Green for Go

Serves 2–3

*1 apple, peeled, cored and
  quartered*
*150 g (5 oz) seedless white
  grapes*

*25 g (1 oz) fresh coriander,
  stalks included*
25 g (1 oz) watercress
1 tbsp fresh lime juice

Place the apple, grapes, coriander and watercress in a blender and mix. Stir in the lime juice and pour into glasses.

Mint Tea

Makes 10–12 glasses (2.25 litres/4 pints)

2.25 l (4 pints) filtered water
100 g (4 oz) mint leaves

Boil the water, then pour it over the leaves in a heatproof bowl. Allow to stand for 15 minutes. Strain, to remove leaves, then pour the tea into cups. Drink hot or cold, with ice. Ideally, you should drink all of this during the course of a couple of days, keeping it in the fridge and throwing away any left after that time.

Apple Mint

Makes 3 glasses (750 ml/1¼ pints)

2 peppermint teabags
175 ml (6 fl oz) boiling filtered water
600 ml (1 pint) apple juice

Place the teabags in the boiling water and allow to stand for 15 minutes. Add the apple juice, allow to cool, then chill in the refrigerator. Serve chilled and drink during the course of a day. For those on the detoxification programme only.

Ginger Tea

Makes 3–4 glasses (850 ml/30 fl oz)

850 ml (30 fl oz) filtered water
4-cm (1.5-in) length fresh ginger root
6–8 catnip teabags
fruit juice sweetener, to taste

Place the water and ginger root in a saucepan and bring to the boil. Cover and simmer for 5 minutes. Remove from the heat, add the teabags and allow to stand for 5 minutes. Remove the teabags. Strain the ginger from the remaining liquid and add fruit juice sweetener to taste. Serve warm or chilled, over ice.

Spicy Pineapple Tea

Serves 5

*350 ml (12 fl oz) pineapple
  juice
350 ml (12 fl oz) filtered water*

*1 tsp whole cloves
2 cinnamon sticks
1 lemon, sliced*

Place the pineapple juice and water in a saucepan and bring to the boil. Add the cloves, cinnamon and lemon slices and reduce the heat. Cover and simmer for 10 minutes. Remove the cloves and cinnamon before serving hot.

Strawberry Delight

Makes 2–3 glasses

*75 g (3 oz) strawberries
175–250 ml (6–8 fl oz) orange
  juice*

*1 small banana
1 tsp fructose
6 ice cubes*

Place all the ingredients in a blender and mix until smooth. Serve immediately.

Rice Tea

Serves 2–3

2 tbsp brown rice
600 ml (1 pint) boiling filtered water
½ tsp honey (optional)

Place the rice in a small, heavy bottomed frying pan over a medium heat. Stir the grains until they give out a roasted aroma. Transfer the rice to a small saucepan, add the boiling water and simmer for 1 minute. Cover and turn off the heat. Allow the tea to steep for 3 minutes. Strain and serve hot, with honey, if using.

Fruit Smoothie

Serves 1

1 banana, cut into chunks
100 g (4 oz) strawberries
50–85 ml (2–3 fl oz) soya milk
* or orange juice*

pinch ground cinnamon
1–2 ice cubes

Place all the ingredients in a blender and mix until smooth. Serve.

Cran-apple Tea

Serves 4

*300 ml (10 fl oz) cranberry
  juice*
300 ml (10 fl oz) filtered water
*4 herbal teabags (peppermint,
  cinnamon, apple, lemon and
  ginger or other flavour of your
  choice)*

4 cinnamon sticks
2 tsp honey or to taste

Pour the cranberry juice and water into a medium saucepan and bring to the boil. Add the teabags and cinnamon sticks. Remove from the heat, cover and steep for 5 minutes. Place a cinnamon stick in each of 4 warmed mugs. Pour the tea into the mugs and add honey to taste.

Banarrot Juice

Serves 3–4

1 ripe banana, sliced
*2 apples, peeled, cored and
  chopped*

4 large carrots, chopped
2 ice cubes (optional)
50 ml (2 fl oz) apple juice

Place all the ingredients in a blender and mix until smooth. Serve.

Banana Milkshake

Serves 1

1 banana, peeled and chopped
*75 g (3 oz) soft fruit, such as
  strawberries or raspberries*

*125-ml (4 fl-oz) carton live
  natural yogurt*
4–8 tbsp semi-skimmed milk

Place the fruit and yogurt in a blender and mix until smooth. Gradually add the milk until the desired consistency is reached. Serve.

References

1 K. J. Pezke, A. Elsner, J. Proll, F. Thielecke and C. C. Metges (2000) *Journal of Nutrition*, **130**, pp. 2889–96.

2 A team of Japanese researchers, led by Dr Yoshiaki Somekawa. See (January 2001) 'Obstetrics and Gynecology' newsletter, **97**,1.

3 J. Kleijnen et al. (November 1992) *Lancet*, **340**, 1136–9.

4 D. Warot (1991) 'Comparative Effects of Ginkgo Biloba Extracts on Psychomotor Performance and Memory in Healthy Subjects', *Therapie*, 46.

5 I. J. Russell, J. E. Michalek, J. D. Flechas and G. E. Abraham (1992) 'Management of Fibromyalgia: Rationale for the use of magnesium and malic acid', *Journal of Nutritional Medicine*, **3**, pp. 49–59.

6 I. J. Russell, J. E. Michalek, J. D. Flechas and G. E. Abraham (1995) 'Treatment of FMS with Supermalic: A randomized, double-blind, placebo-controlled crossover pilot study', *Journal of Rheumatology*, **22**, pp. 953–8.

Useful addresses

General

The American Fibromyalgia Syndrome Association
PO Box 32698
Tucson
AZ 85751
USA
Tel.: 520 733 1570
Website: www.afsafund.org

FibroAction
Tel.: 0844 443 5422
Website: www.fibroaction.org

This charitable organization provides information about fibromyalgia, and has a good social media team to help and support people, mainly online.

The Fibromyalgia Association UK
Studio 3007, Mile End Mill
12 Seedhill Road
Paisley PA1 1JS
Tel.: 0844 826 9022 (general enquiries, not for support)
Helpline: 0844 887 2444 (10 a.m. to 4 p.m., Monday to Friday)
Website: www.fmauk.org

A registered charity administered by volunteers and established to provide information and support to those with the condition and their families. In addition the Association provides medical information for professionals, a patient-information pack and a magazine, *Fibromyalgia Focus*. The website contains a community forum.

The Fibromyalgia Network
PO Box 31750
Tucson
AZ 85751
USA
Tel.: 800 853 2929
Website: www.fmnetnews.com

For quarterly newsletters, information and advice. You can email the network directly from the website.

Fibromyalgia Support Northern Ireland
PO Box 293
Bangor BT20 9AQ
Tel.: 028 9127 1525
Helpline: 0844 826 9024 (10.30 a.m. to 4 p.m., Monday to Friday)
Text: 08448 269024 (for urgent enquiries when out and about: no
abbreviations please)
Website: www.fmsni.org.uk

This organization is dedicated to raising fibromyalgia awareness and
supporting people with fibromyalgia. Drop-in services are available in
Belfast and Coleraine.

National Fibromyalgia Association
1000 Bristol Street, North Suite 17–247,
Newport Beach
CA 92660
USA
Website: www.fmaware.org

The members-only website provides an online store and chatroom and
gives information on support groups and FM community events from
Canada to California. The monthly *Fibromyalgia AWARE* magazine (at
present *The New! Fibromyalgia AWARE Magazine*) may be received online or
in a printed version by subscription.

UK Fibromyalgia
7 Ashbourne Road
Bournemouth BH5 2JS
Tel. and Fax: 01202 259155
Website: www.ukfibromyalgia.com

For fibromyalgia information and advice, experts' comments and more.
Providers of the monthly *Fibromyalgia* magazine.

Arthritis

Arthritis Care
Floor 4, Linen Court
10 East Road
London N1 6AD
Tel.: 020 7380 6500
Helpline: 0808 800 4050 (free, 10 a.m. to 4 p.m., Monday to Friday)
Website: www.arthritiscare.org.uk

The website provides details of other regional and national offices in
the UK.

Arthritis Research UK
Copeman House
St Mary's Court
St Mary's Gate
Chesterfield S41 7TD
Tel.: 0300 790 0400
Website: www.arthritisresearchuk.org

Water filters and seasonings

Enzyme Process UK
7 The Flaxmill
Flaxmill Lane
Pinchbeck
Spalding
Lincolnshire
PE11 3YP

Tel.: 0845 1300 776

For high-performance fresh water filters.

Nutritional supplement specialists

Bioforce
Helpline: 0845 608 5858 (8.30 a.m. to 5 p.m., Monday to Saturday)
Website: www.avogel.co.uk
Markets A. Vogel health remedies.

Blue Green Planet
5 Adelaide Park
Belfast BT9 6FX
Northern Ireland

Fax: 02890 661577
Website: www.bluegreenplanet.co.uk

Upper Klamath algae contains all the required nutrients, plus many powerful antioxidants to aid detoxification.

Total Wellbeing Solutions Ltd
Unit 12, Trident Industrial Estate
Blackthorne Road
Colnbrook SL3 0AX

Tel.: 01753 287877
Website: www.totalwellbeingsolutions.co.uk

For an excellent one-a-day high antioxidant containing over 30 ingredients including the B vitamins and high-dose pantothenic acid, and omega 3 and omega 6 essential fatty acids (which help to control pain and inflammation), Liver Support (which gets the liver and gall bladder working properly so that toxins are expelled) and Intestinal Tone (which balances the gut flora and removes toxins from the body, helping to ease constipation or diarrhoea, flatulence and bloating).

Vanderbell Health
32 Collyer Avenue
Beddington
Surrey CRO 4QU

Tel.: 020 8680 2888 (24-hour order line)
Website: www.health4youonline.com

For magnesium malate (which helps to reduce the pain and fatigue of fibromyalgia) and SucroGuard (which helps reduce food and cigarette cravings) and all other high-quality nutritional supplements.

Vitamins Direct Ltd
PO Box 621
York House
Wetherby Road
York YO26 0EX

Tel.: 0800 634 9985 (free, 9 a.m. to 6 p.m., Monday to Saturday)
Website: http://vitaminsdirectonline.co.uk

For glucosamine, co-enzyme Q10, ginkgo biloba, evening primrose oil and the B complex vitamins.

Further reading

Stephen J. Barrett and Ronald E. Gots (1998) *Chemical Sensitivity*, Prometheus Books.

Christine Craggs-Hinton (2014) *Living with Fibromyalgia*, third edition, Sheldon Press.

Christine Craggs-Hinton (2006) *How to Beat Pain: Techniques that work*, Sheldon Press

Andrew Hall Cutler (1999) *Amalgam Illness, Diagnosis and Treatment*, Minerva Laboratories.

Stephen Edelson (1998) *Living with Environmental Illness*, Taylor Publishing Company.

Joe Fitzgibbon (1993) *Feeling Tired All The Time*, Gill and Macmillan.

Mary Moeller and Karl Moeller (1997) *Fibromyalgia Cookbook*, Fibromyalgia Solutions.

Barry Sears (1999) *The Zone Diet*, HarperCollins.

Shelley Ann Velekei (2000) *The Fibromyalgia Recipe Book*, Smith Velekei Publishing.

Index

5-Hydroxytryptophan (5-HTP) 28, 43

additives 7, 13, 50, 55–6, 60; *see also individual additives*
adrenal glands 35, 45, 50
alcohol 73, 77, 79
aluminium 43, 57, 60
amalgam tooth fillings 29, 61
amino acids 18, 27–8
antibodies 29, 61
antioxidants 14, 23, 30–1, 53
aspartame 10, 13, 54–5, 56

B complex vitamins 33–6, 41, 48; *see also individual vitamins*
biotin 38–9
blood sugar 22, 25
boron 44, 48
butylated hydroxyanisole (BHT) 55

caffeine 13, 25, 50–1
calcium 11, 15, 36, 40, 44, 48
carbohydrates 12, 15–22
central nervous system 6, 8, 41, 53, 59, 60
chelation 39
chemical pesticides 6, 7, 9, 22, 53, 62, 64, 65
chemical sensitivities 58–9
cholesterol 18, 24
chromium 43
cider vinegar 67, 68–9
coconut oil 67–8
coeliac disease 10–11
cortisol 6, 29

dairy products 10, 15, 18, 71–2
detoxification 14, 29, 53, 57, ch. 7; superfoods 64–7
DHEA (dehydroepiandrosterone) 45
digestive enzymes 8, 18
diuretics 25

eggs 18–19, 24
electro-acupuncture 28
endocrine system 6, 8, 59
exercise 9, 60, 77, 79

fat: polyunsaturated 12, 15, 23; saturated 13, 16, 18, 22–4; unsaturated 12, 15–17, 23–4
fatty acids 22, 23, 30, 67, 68
fibre 13, 17, 24–5
fibromyalgia: causes 5–6; diagnosis 5; 'flare-up' of symptoms 4; genetic factors in 4, 29; symptoms 3–4
food: intake diary, keeping 72; junk/ fast 7–8, 13, 17, 41, 56, 72, 79; sensitivities 9–11; *see also* dairy products, eggs, fruit, main meals, soups, soya products
free radicals 23, 30–1
fresh air 79
fruit 11, 12, 13, 15, 17, 20, 21, 22, 64–5

ginkgo biloba 38, 45, 48
gluten intolerance 10–11
glucosamine 44, 48
guaifenesin 70

insulin 21, 22, 34, 42, 51
irritable bowel syndrome 3, 10–11, 25, 37, 59

junk foods/fast foods *see under* food

lecithin 24

magnesium 15, 35, 39–41, 43, 46–8, 59
magnesium malate 43, 46–7, 48
main meals 95–120
manganese 39, 41, 47–8
menus, suggested 81–2, ch. 7
mercury 29, 61
milk thistle 38, 45, 48, 69

minerals 15, 25, 39–43; *see also*
   individual minerals
monosodium glutamate (MSG) 55

nutritional supplements ch. 5; *see also*
   individual supplements

oil of evening primrose 46, 48
organophosphates 58–60
osteoporosis 14–15, 20, 36, 39, 40,
   44, 45
oxalates 11
oxidative stress 19, 30, 48

potassium 41, 65
proanthocyanidins 30, 38
protein 13, 16, 17, 18–20

salicylates 70–1
selenium 30, 42
serotonin 5–6, 28, 33, 35, 43
sleep 3, 5, 28, 29, 37, 43, 74, 78
smoking 13, 31, 32, 50, 53–4, 61
sorbate 55
soups 91–4
soya products 20–1
spices 69–70; *see also* turmeric
stimulants 50–5
stress 4, 6, 28, 29, 35, 38, 39, 50

sugar 51–3
surgery 6, 28, 32, 70

thyroid 3, 10, 21, 28, 34,
   59, 74
Transcutaneous Electrical Nerve
   Stimulation (TENS) 28
tryptophan 28
turmeric 30, 69–70
tyrosine 28

viral illness 6
vitamin D deficiency 37
vitamins: A (beta-carotene) 32–3; B1
   (thiamine) 33–4; B2 (riboflavin)
   34; B3 (niacinamide) 34–5;
   B5 (pantothenic acid) 35; B6
   (pyridoxine) 35; B12 (cobalamin)
   35–6; C (ascorbic acid) 32; D 36–7;
   E 33; P 38

water: distilled 57, 75; filtered 13,
   57–8, 61, 64
water filters 57
weight 54–5, 68, 73–5
whiplash 6
World Health Organization 17

zinc 42